Conquering Head and Neck Cancer

Treatment, Recovery and Life After Diagnosis

Isabella White

Copyright © 2023 by Isabella White.

Disclaimer: The information contained in this book is based on the research, opinions, and experiences of the author. It is not intended to replace professional medical advice or treatment. The reader should regularly consult a physician for any health issues and always seek the advice of a physician before modifying diet, supplement, or exercise regimens.

The author and publisher shall have neither liability nor responsibility to any person or entity concerning any loss or damage related to the information contained in this book. The information provided is general in nature and may not apply to every individual. Any reliance on the information contained herein is solely at the reader's own risk.

Contents

Introduction

Receiving a head and neck cancer diagnosis can feel devastating. Whether it's a tumor in the oral cavity, throat, larynx, sinuses, or nasal cavity, facing the upcoming treatment and its effects is frightening and uncertain.

This book provides the comprehensive guide that patients need when starting their cancer journey. It equips readers with the knowledge to take an active role in their care throughout the process.

Covering everything from the various types and risk factors to emerging treatments and life after recovery, this book will serve as a support system and resource manual. It explains head and neck cancers in an easy-to-understand way and outlines both established and new therapies, from surgery and chemotherapy to immunotherapy.

Just as importantly, this book covers what happens after treatment ends. From remission to potential recurrence, readers will learn how to navigate follow-up care, physical and emotional issues, and return slowly to everyday life.

Additional guidance is provided on support networks, communicating with loved ones, nutrition, and more.

This book complements doctors' expertise by empowering patients to advocate for their needs, understand options fully, and cope through every phase.

Together, we will tackle each challenge with knowledge, hope, and clarity so that patients can focus on healing and thriving. Let's begin the journey.

Chapter 1

Understanding Head and Neck Cancer

What is Head and Neck Cancer?

Head and neck cancer refers to a group of cancers that develop in the region of the head and neck. This includes cancers that affect various parts such as the mouth, throat, nose, sinuses, salivary glands, and lymph nodes in the neck. These cancers can occur in different areas of the head and neck, including the oral cavity, larynx, pharynx, and nasal cavity.

Cancer occurs when the cells in the body grow and divide uncontrollably, forming a mass of abnormal cells called a tumor. In the case of head and neck cancer, these tumors can interfere with the normal functioning of the affected areas, leading to a range of symptoms and complications.

There are several different types of head and neck cancer, each with its own characteristics and treatment options. The most common type is squamous cell carcinoma, which develops in the squamous cells that line the mucosal surfaces of the head and neck. Other less common types include salivary gland tumors, thyroid cancer, and nasopharyngeal cancer.

Head and neck cancer is a disease that can affect anyone, but there are certain factors that can increase the risk of developing it. The leading causes of head and neck cancer are tobacco and alcohol use, particularly in the oral cavity and larynx. In addition to this, human papillomavirus (HPV) infection is also a significant risk factor for certain types of head and neck cancer, especially in the oropharynx.

The signs and symptoms of head and neck cancer can vary depending on the location and stage of the disease. Common symptoms include a persistent sore throat, difficulty swallowing, hoarseness, a lump or sore that doesn't heal, and changes in voice or speech. Other symptoms may include ear pain, facial numbness, and unexplained weight loss.

Early detection is crucial for the successful treatment of head and neck cancer. Regular self-examinations and routine check-ups with a healthcare professional can help identify any abnormalities or warning signs. If a potential issue is detected, further diagnostic tests, such as imaging scans and biopsies, may be performed to confirm the diagnosis.

Once a diagnosis of head and neck cancer is confirmed, the stage of the disease will be determined. Staging helps determine the extent of the cancer and guides treatment decisions. The stages range from I to IV, with stage I being the earliest and stage IV being the most advanced.

Treatment options for head and neck cancer depend on various factors, including the type, stage, and location of the cancer, as well as the overall health of the patient. The main treatment modalities include surgery, radiation therapy, chemotherapy, and targeted therapy. In some cases, a combination of these treatments may be used to achieve the best possible outcome.

Surgery is often the primary treatment for localized head and neck cancer. It involves removing the tumor and any affected surrounding tissues. Depending on the location and size of the tumor, reconstructive surgery may be necessary to restore the appearance and function of the affected area.

Radiation therapy uses high-energy beams to kill cancer cells and shrink tumors. It can be used as the primary treatment or in combination with surgery or chemotherapy. Chemotherapy involves the use of drugs to kill cancer cells throughout the body, while targeted therapy specifically targets cancer cells by blocking the signals that allow them to grow and divide.

In addition to these treatments, supportive care and rehabilitation play a crucial role in the overall management of head and neck cancer. Supportive care focuses on managing the side effects of treatment and improving the quality of life for patients. Rehabilitation helps patients regain their speech, swallowing, and other functions affected by the cancer and its treatment.

In the next section, we will delve deeper into the various types and stages of head and neck cancer, providing a comprehensive understanding of the disease and its implications. Understanding the specifics of your diagnosis is essential for making informed decisions about your treatment and recovery journey.

Types and Stages of Head and Neck Cancer

The mouth, throat, nose, sinuses, salivary glands, and lymph nodes are just a few of the complex organs in the head and neck that can be affected by cancer. Understanding the different types and stages of head and neck cancer is crucial in determining the most appropriate treatment plan and predicting the prognosis.

Types of Head and Neck Cancer

There are various types of head and neck cancer, each of which develops from distinct tissues and cells in the head and neck region. The most common types include:

1. **Squamous cell carcinoma:** This is the most common type of head and neck cancer, accounting for roughly 90% of all cases. It typically develops in the lining of the mouth, throat, or voice box.

2. **Salivary gland tumors:** These tumors originate in the salivary glands, which produce saliva. There are three main types of salivary gland tumors: mucoepidermoid carcinoma, adenoid cystic carcinoma, and adenocarcinoma.

3. **Nasopharyngeal carcinoma:** This type of cancer arises in the nasopharynx, the upper part of the

throat behind the nose. It is more common in certain regions, such as Southeast Asia.

4. **Laryngeal cancer:** Laryngeal cancer affects the voice box (larynx) and can cause changes in voice, difficulty swallowing, or a persistent cough.

5. **Oropharyngeal cancer:** This type of cancer develops in the oropharynx, which includes the back of the throat, base of the tongue, and tonsils. It is often associated with a human papillomavirus (HPV) infection.

6. **Hypopharyngeal cancer:** Hypopharyngeal cancer occurs in the hypopharynx, the lower part of the throat. It is often diagnosed at an advanced stage due to its location and lack of early symptoms.

7. **Sinus and nasal cavity cancer:** These cancers develop in the sinuses or nasal cavity and can cause symptoms such as nasal congestion, facial pain, or frequent sinus infections.

Stages of Head and Neck Cancer

Once a diagnosis of head and neck cancer is made, it is important to determine the stage of the disease. Staging helps in understanding the extent of cancer spread and guides treatment decisions. The stages of head and neck cancer are typically classified using the TNM system, which stands for Tumor, Node, and Metastasis.

1. **Tumor (T) stage:** The T stage describes the size and extent of the primary tumor. It ranges from T0 (no evidence of a primary tumor) to T4 (a large tumor that has invaded nearby structures).

2. **Node (N) stage:** The N stage indicates whether the cancer has spread to nearby lymph nodes. It ranges from N0 (no lymph node involvement) to N3 (extensive lymph node involvement).

3. **Metastasis (M) stage:** The M stage determines whether the cancer has spread to distant parts of the body. It is classified as M0 (no distant metastasis) or M1 (distant metastasis present).

Head and neck cancer is further divided into stages, from stage 0 (carcinoma in situ) to stage IV (advanced cancer with distant metastasis), based on the combination of T, N, and M stages.

It is important to note that the specific staging system may vary depending on the type of head and neck cancer. For example, laryngeal cancer has its own staging system known as the TNM staging system for laryngeal cancer.

Understanding the stage of head and neck cancer is crucial, as it helps healthcare professionals determine the most appropriate treatment options and predict the prognosis. Treatment options may include surgery, radiation therapy, chemotherapy, targeted therapy, or a combination of these approaches.

In the next section, we will explore the causes and risk factors associated with head and neck cancer, shedding light on the factors that may increase an individual's susceptibility to developing this disease.

Causes and Risk Factors

Head and neck cancer can be caused by a variety of factors, both controllable and uncontrollable. Understanding these causes and risk factors can help you make informed decisions about your lifestyle and reduce your chances of developing this disease. While it's important to remember that not everyone who has these risk factors will develop head and neck cancer, being aware of them can still be beneficial.

Tobacco and Alcohol Use

One of the most significant risk factors for head and neck cancer is the use of tobacco products, including cigarettes, cigars, and smokeless tobacco. Smoking tobacco not only increases the risk of developing cancer in the lungs but also in the head and neck region.

Similarly, excessive alcohol consumption is also strongly associated with an increased risk of head and neck cancer. The risk is even higher for individuals who both smoke and drink heavily.

Human Papillomavirus (HPV) Infection

In recent years, the prevalence of head and neck cancer caused by human papillomavirus (HPV) infection has been on the rise. HPV is a sexually transmitted infection that can lead to the development of certain types of head and neck cancers, particularly in the oropharynx (the middle part of the throat). It's important to note that not all HPV infections lead to cancer, but certain strains of the virus, such as HPV-16, are more strongly associated with the development of head and neck cancer.

Poor Oral Hygiene

Maintaining good oral hygiene is not only important for preventing cavities and gum disease but also for reducing the risk of head and neck cancer. Poor oral hygiene can lead to chronic inflammation and infection in the mouth, which can increase the risk of developing cancer. Regular dental check-ups, proper brushing and flossing, and avoiding tobacco and excessive alcohol use are all essential for maintaining good oral health.

Occupational Exposure

Certain occupations and work environments can expose individuals to substances that increase the risk of head and neck cancer. For example, individuals who work in industries such as construction, mining, or manufacturing may be exposed to chemicals, dust, or fumes that can irritate the lining of the throat and increase the risk of cancer. Individuals in these professions need to take appropriate safety precautions and follow recommended guidelines to minimize their exposure to these harmful substances.

Age and Gender

Head and neck cancer can occur at any age, but it is more commonly diagnosed in individuals over the age of 50. Additionally, men are more likely to develop head and neck cancer than women.

The reasons for these differences are not fully understood, but hormonal and lifestyle factors may play a role. Regardless of age or gender, everyone needs to be aware of the risk factors and take steps to reduce their chances of developing this disease.

Genetic Factors

While most head and neck cancers are not directly caused by inherited genetic mutations, certain genetic factors can increase an individual's susceptibility to developing the disease. For example, individuals with a family history of head and neck cancer may have a higher risk of developing the disease themselves.

Additionally, certain genetic conditions, such as Fanconi anemia, are associated with an increased risk of head and neck cancer. If you have a family history of head and neck cancer or a known genetic condition, it's important to discuss this with your healthcare provider.

Other Risk Factors

Several other risk factors have been associated with an increased risk of head and neck cancer, although the evidence is not as strong as for the factors mentioned above. These include:

- **Poor nutrition:** A diet lacking in fruits and vegetables may increase the risk of developing head and neck cancer.

- **Chronic acid reflux:** Long-term acid reflux can cause chronic irritation and inflammation in the throat, which may increase the risk of cancer.

- **Weakened immune system:** Individuals with weakened immune systems, such as those with HIV/AIDS or who have undergone organ transplantation, may have a higher risk of developing head and neck cancer.

- **Sun exposure:** Prolonged exposure to the sun's ultraviolet (UV) rays can increase the risk of lip cancer.

It's important to remember that having one or more of these risk factors does not mean that you will develop head and neck cancer. Conversely, not having any of these risk factors does not guarantee that you will not develop the disease. However, being aware of these risk factors can help you make informed decisions about your lifestyle and take steps to reduce your risk.

Signs and Symptoms

Recognizing the signs and symptoms of head and neck cancer is crucial for early detection and successful treatment. While the specific symptoms can vary depending on the location and stage of the cancer, there are some common signs to be aware of.

It's important to remember that experiencing one or more of these symptoms does not necessarily mean you have cancer, but it's always best to consult with a healthcare professional if you have any concerns.

Common Symptoms

1. **Persistent sore throat:** If you have a sore throat that lasts for more than two weeks and doesn't seem to improve with over-the-counter remedies, it's worth getting it checked out. While a sore throat can be caused by many factors, including viral infections, allergies, or acid reflux, it can also be a symptom of head and neck cancer.

2. **Difficulty swallowing:** Difficulty or pain while swallowing, also known as dysphagia, can be a sign of head and neck cancer. This symptom may be accompanied by a feeling of a lump or obstruction in the throat or neck.

3. **Voice changes:** Hoarseness or a persistent change in your voice that lasts for more than two weeks should not be ignored. It can be a result of vocal

cord involvement or other structures in the head and neck area.

4. **Unexplained weight loss:** If you are losing weight without trying or experiencing a significant loss of appetite, it could be a sign of head and neck cancer. Unexplained weight loss is often associated with advanced stages of the disease.

5. **Swelling or lumps:** Any unexplained swelling or lumps in the neck, throat, or mouth should be evaluated by a healthcare professional. These lumps may be painless or tender to the touch.

6. **Persistent ear pain:** Head and neck cancers can sometimes cause referred pain to the ears. If you have persistent ear pain that is not related to an ear infection or other known cause, it's important to have it checked out.

7. **Numbness or weakness:** Numbness or weakness in the face, neck, or other areas of the head can be a symptom of certain types of head and neck cancer. This symptom may be accompanied by difficulty moving the affected area.

8. **Persistent nasal congestion or sinus problems:** Chronic nasal congestion or sinus issues that do not respond to usual treatments may be a sign of head

and neck cancer, particularly if accompanied by other symptoms such as nosebleeds or facial pain.

9. **Bleeding:** Unexplained bleeding from the mouth, nose, or throat should be evaluated by a healthcare professional. While there can be various causes for bleeding, it's important to rule out head and neck cancer as a potential cause.

10. **Skin changes:** Skin changes, such as ulcers, sores, or discoloration on the face, neck, or scalp, should not be ignored. These changes can sometimes be a sign of skin cancer or other types of head and neck cancer.

Less Common Symptoms

In addition to the common symptoms mentioned above, there are some less common signs and symptoms that may indicate head and neck cancer. These include:

- **Persistent cough:** A chronic cough that doesn't go away or worsens over time can be a symptom of certain types of head and neck cancer, such as laryngeal or lung cancer.

- **Difficulty breathing:** If you experience difficulty breathing or shortness of breath, it's important to seek medical attention. While this symptom can be caused by various factors, it can also be a sign of advanced head and neck cancer.

- **Changes in vision or hearing:** In some cases, head and neck cancers can affect the nerves responsible for vision or hearing, leading to changes in these senses. If you notice any changes in your vision or hearing, it's important to have them evaluated.

- **Persistent headaches:** While headaches are a common ailment, persistent or severe headaches that are not relieved by usual treatments should be investigated further.

- **Unexplained facial pain:** Facial pain that is not related to a known cause, such as dental issues or sinus problems, should be evaluated by a healthcare professional.

- **Difficulty opening the mouth:** If you experience difficulty opening your mouth fully or have limited jaw movement, it could be a sign of head and neck cancer, particularly if accompanied by other symptoms.

Remember, these symptoms can be caused by various factors, and having one or more of them does not necessarily mean you have head and neck cancer. However, if you experience any persistent or concerning symptoms, it's important to consult with a healthcare professional for a proper evaluation and diagnosis. Early detection and treatment can greatly improve the chances of successful outcomes in head and neck cancer.

Chapter 2

Diagnosis and Treatment Options

Diagnosing Head and Neck Cancer

Diagnosing head and neck cancer is a crucial step in the journey toward conquering this disease. Early detection plays a significant role in improving treatment outcomes and increasing the chances of a successful recovery. In this section, we will explore the various methods and procedures used to diagnose head and neck cancer, providing you with a comprehensive understanding of what to expect during the diagnostic process.

Clinical Evaluation

The first step in diagnosing head and neck cancer is a thorough clinical evaluation. Your healthcare provider will begin by taking a detailed medical history, including any symptoms you may be experiencing and any risk factors that may be present. They will also perform a physical examination, focusing on the head and neck region, to check for any abnormalities or signs of cancer.

During the physical examination, your healthcare provider may examine your mouth, throat, and neck, feeling for any lumps or enlarged lymph nodes. They may also use a small mirror or a flexible tube with a camera (an endoscope) to visualize the inside of your throat and other areas of concern. This examination allows them to assess the extent of the disease and determine the next steps in the diagnostic process.

Imaging Tests

Imaging tests are commonly used to further evaluate and diagnose head and neck cancer. These tests provide detailed images of the affected areas, helping healthcare professionals identify the location, size, and spread of the tumor. Some of the most commonly used imaging tests include:

- **X-rays:** X-rays are a simple and non-invasive imaging technique that uses low levels of radiation to create images of the inside of your body. While they may not provide as much detail as other imaging tests, they can be useful in identifying abnormalities in the bones of the head and neck.

- **Computed Tomography (CT) Scan:** A CT scan combines multiple X-ray images to create detailed cross-sectional images of the head and neck. This imaging technique provides a more comprehensive view of the affected areas, allowing healthcare professionals to assess the size and location of the tumor as well as any spread to nearby lymph nodes or other structures.

- **Magnetic Resonance Imaging (MRI):** An MRI uses a powerful magnetic field and radio waves to create detailed images of the soft tissues in the head and neck. This imaging technique is particularly useful in evaluating the extent of the tumor and determining if it has spread to nearby structures, such as the brain or blood vessels.

- **Positron Emission Tomography (PET) Scan**: A PET scan involves injecting a small amount of radioactive material into your body, which is then detected by a special camera. This test can help identify areas of increased metabolic activity, which may indicate the presence of cancer cells. PET scans are often used in combination with CT scans to provide a more accurate assessment of the tumor and its spread.

Biopsy

A biopsy is the definitive diagnostic test for head and neck cancer. It involves the removal of a small sample of tissue from the affected area, which is then examined under a microscope by a pathologist. The biopsy helps determine the type of cancer, its grade, and whether it has spread to nearby tissues or lymph nodes.

Different types of biopsies can be performed, depending on the location and size of the tumor. Some common biopsy techniques include:

- **Fine Needle Aspiration (FNA) Biopsy:** An FNA biopsy involves inserting a thin needle into the tumor to extract a small sample of cells. This procedure is often used for tumors located in the neck or lymph nodes.
- **Incisional Biopsy:** An incisional biopsy involves surgically removing a small portion of the tumor for examination. This type of biopsy is typically performed when the tumor is large or located in a difficult-to-access area.
- **Excisional Biopsy:** An excisional biopsy involves surgically removing the entire tumor along with a margin of healthy tissue. This type of biopsy is

usually performed when the tumor is small and easily accessible.

Additional Tests

In some cases, additional tests may be necessary to further evaluate the extent of the disease and plan the most appropriate treatment. These tests may include:

- **Blood Tests:** Blood tests can help assess your overall health and detect any abnormalities that may be associated with head and neck cancer. They can also provide information about the function of your organs, such as the liver and kidneys, which may be affected by the disease or its treatment.

- **Molecular Testing:** Molecular testing involves analyzing the genetic material of the tumor cells to identify specific genetic mutations or alterations. This information can help guide treatment decisions and determine the prognosis of the disease.

- **Lymph Node Evaluation:** If there is suspicion of lymph node involvement, a procedure called a sentinel lymph node biopsy may be performed. This involves injecting a dye or radioactive substance near the tumor to identify the first lymph node(s) that the cancer is likely to spread to. These lymph nodes can then be removed and examined for the presence of cancer cells.

The Importance of a Multidisciplinary Approach

Diagnosing head and neck cancer requires a multidisciplinary team of healthcare professionals, including otolaryngologists, oncologists, radiologists, and pathologists. These specialists work together to ensure an accurate diagnosis and develop an individualized treatment plan tailored to your specific needs.

Remember, early detection is key in the fight against head and neck cancer. If you experience any persistent symptoms or notice any changes in your head and neck region, it is important to seek medical attention promptly. By understanding the diagnostic process and working closely with your healthcare team, you can take an active role in your journey towards conquering head and neck cancer.

Medical Imaging and Biopsy

Medical imaging and biopsy are crucial steps in the diagnosis and staging of head and neck cancer. These procedures help doctors gather essential information about the location, size, and extent of the tumor, as well as determine the most appropriate treatment plan for each individual. In this section, we will explore the different types of medical imaging techniques used in the diagnosis of head and neck cancer, as well as the importance of a biopsy in confirming the presence of cancer cells.

Medical Imaging Techniques

Medical imaging plays a vital role in the initial assessment and diagnosis of head and neck cancer. It allows doctors to visualize the affected area and identify any abnormalities or tumors. There are several imaging techniques commonly used in the evaluation of head and neck cancer:

1. **X-rays:** X-rays are a commonly used imaging technique that can provide a basic overview of the affected area. They can help identify bone abnormalities, such as fractures or erosion, and detect the presence of tumors. However, X-rays may not provide detailed information about soft tissues, making them less effective in diagnosing certain types of head and neck cancer.

2. **Computed Tomography (CT) Scan:** A CT scan is a more advanced imaging technique that uses X-rays and computer technology to create detailed cross-sectional images of the head and neck. It

provides a more comprehensive view of the affected area, allowing doctors to assess the size, location, and extent of the tumor. CT scans are particularly useful in detecting tumors in the throat, larynx, and sinuses.

3. **Magnetic Resonance Imaging (MRI):** MRI uses a powerful magnetic field and radio waves to produce detailed images of the head and neck. It provides excellent visualization of soft tissues, making it particularly useful in detecting tumors in the tongue, tonsils, and salivary glands. MRI can also help determine the involvement of nearby structures and lymph nodes.

4. **Positron Emission Tomography (PET) Scan:** PET scans involve the injection of a small amount of radioactive material into the body. This material is absorbed by cancer cells, which can then be detected by a special camera. PET scans are useful in determining the metabolic activity of tumors and identifying areas of cancer spread, such as lymph nodes or distant metastases. They are often combined with CT scans to provide more accurate staging information.

Biopsy

While medical imaging techniques can provide valuable information about the presence and location of tumors, a biopsy is necessary to confirm the diagnosis of head and neck cancer. During a biopsy, a small sample of tissue is taken from the affected area and examined under a microscope to determine if cancer cells are present.

Different types of biopsies can be performed depending on the location and size of the tumor:

1. **Fine Needle Aspiration (FNA) Biopsy:** An FNA biopsy is a minimally invasive procedure that involves inserting a thin needle into the tumor to extract a small sample of cells. This type of biopsy is commonly used for tumors located in the neck or lymph nodes. An FNA biopsy is relatively quick and can be performed in an outpatient setting.

2. **Incisional Biopsy:** An incisional biopsy involves the removal of a small piece of the tumor for examination. This type of biopsy is typically performed when the tumor is large or located in a difficult-to-access area. It may require local or general anesthesia, depending on the location and size of the tumor.

3. **Excisional Biopsy:** An excisional biopsy involves the complete removal of the tumor along with a margin of healthy tissue. This type of biopsy is often performed when the tumor is small and easily accessible. It may require local or general anesthesia, depending on the location and size of the tumor.

4. **Endoscopic Biopsy:** An endoscopic biopsy is performed using a thin, flexible tube with a camera and a light source called an endoscope. The endoscope is inserted through the mouth or nose to visualize and biopsy tumors located in the throat, larynx, or esophagus. This type of biopsy is minimally invasive and can be performed on an outpatient basis.

Once the biopsy sample is obtained, it is sent to a pathologist, who examines the tissue under a microscope. The pathologist will determine if cancer cells are present and provide additional information about the type and grade of the tumor. This information is crucial in determining the most appropriate treatment plan for each individual.

Surgical Treatment Options

Surgery is one of the primary treatment options for head and neck cancer. It involves the removal of the tumor and surrounding tissues to eliminate the cancer cells. The specific surgical procedure recommended will depend on the location, size, and stage of the tumor, as well as the overall health of the patient. In this section, we will explore the different surgical treatment options available for head and neck cancer.

1. Primary Tumor Resection

Primary tumor resection is the most common surgical procedure for head and neck cancer. It involves the removal of the tumor and a margin of healthy tissue surrounding it. The goal is to ensure that all cancer cells are removed, reducing the risk of recurrence. The extent of the resection will depend on the size and location of the tumor. In some cases, reconstructive surgery may be necessary to restore the appearance and function of the affected area.

2. Neck Dissection

Neck dissection is a surgical procedure performed to remove lymph nodes in the neck that may be affected by cancer. The lymph nodes are an important part of the body's immune system and can serve as a pathway for cancer cells to spread. During a neck dissection, the surgeon will remove the lymph nodes in the affected area, along with any surrounding tissue that may contain cancer cells. This procedure helps to prevent the spread of cancer and provides valuable information about the stage and extent of the disease.

3. Reconstructive Surgery

Reconstructive surgery is often performed after the removal of a tumor to restore the appearance and function of the affected area. Depending on the location and size of the tumor, reconstructive surgery may involve the use of grafts, flaps, or implants to rebuild the structures that were removed. The goal of reconstructive surgery is to improve the patient's quality of life and help them regain normal functions such as speaking, swallowing, and breathing.

4. Laser Surgery

Laser surgery is a minimally invasive surgical technique that uses a laser beam to remove or destroy cancer cells. It is commonly used for tumors located in the mouth, throat, or larynx. The laser beam can precisely target and remove cancerous tissue while minimizing damage to surrounding healthy tissue. Laser surgery offers several advantages, including reduced bleeding, a shorter recovery time, and improved cosmetic outcomes.

5. Transoral Robotic Surgery (TORS)

Transoral robotic surgery (TORS) is a relatively new surgical technique that uses a robotic system to remove tumors located in the mouth, throat, or larynx. During the procedure, the surgeon controls the robotic arms to access and remove the tumor through the mouth, without the need for external incisions. TORS offers several benefits, including improved precision, reduced scarring, and faster recovery compared to traditional open surgery.

6. Mohs Surgery

Mohs surgery, also known as micrographic surgery, is a specialized surgical technique used to treat skin cancer, including certain types of head and neck cancer. It involves the removal of thin layers of tissue, which are immediately examined under a microscope to check for the presence of cancer cells. This process is repeated until no cancer cells are detected. Mohs surgery offers a high cure rate and minimizes the removal of healthy tissue, making it an effective treatment option for certain types of head and neck cancer.

7. Salvage Surgery

Salvage surgery is performed when cancer recurs or persists after initial treatment, such as radiation therapy or chemotherapy. It involves the removal of the recurrent or persistent tumor, along with any surrounding tissue that may contain cancer cells. Salvage surgery can be challenging due to the potential damage caused by previous treatments. However, it can offer a chance for a cure or long-term control of the disease in select cases.

8. Complications and Risks

Like any surgical procedure, there are potential complications and risks associated with surgical treatment for head and neck cancer. These may include bleeding, infection, damage to nearby structures, changes in appearance or function, and the need for additional surgeries. Patients need to discuss these risks with their healthcare team and understand the potential benefits and drawbacks of each surgical option.

Non-Surgical Treatment Options

When it comes to treating head and neck cancer, surgery is not always the only option. There are several non-surgical treatment options available that can be just as effective in fighting the disease. These treatments may be used alone or in combination with surgery, depending on the specific circumstances of each patient. In this section, we will explore some of the non-surgical treatment options commonly used for head and neck cancer.

1. Radiation Therapy

Radiation therapy, also known as radiotherapy, is a common non-surgical treatment option for head and neck cancer. It kills cancer cells and shrinks tumors by using high-energy X-rays or other types of radiation. Radiation therapy can be administered both externally and internally.

External beam radiation therapy is the most commonly used type of radiation therapy for head and neck cancer. The tumor is targeted using radiation beams from a machine outside the body. The treatment is typically given in daily sessions for several weeks. Each session lasts only a few minutes and is completely painless.

Internal radiation therapy, also referred to as brachytherapy, involves injecting radioactive material into or close to the tumor. This enables a higher dose of radiation to be delivered to cancer cells while minimizing damage to surrounding healthy tissues. Brachytherapy is typically used for smaller tumors or as a boost after external beam radiation therapy.

Radiation therapy can cause side effects such as fatigue, skin changes, difficulty swallowing, and a dry mouth. These side effects are usually temporary and can be managed with the help of your healthcare team. It is important to discuss potential side effects and their management strategies with your healthcare provider before starting radiation therapy.

2. Chemotherapy

Chemotherapy is another non-surgical treatment option that may be used for head and neck cancer. It involves the use of drugs to kill cancer cells throughout the body. Chemotherapy can be given before surgery to shrink tumors, after surgery to kill any remaining cancer cells, or as the primary treatment for advanced or recurrent cancer.

Chemotherapy drugs can be administered orally or intravenously. They travel through the bloodstream, targeting cancer cells wherever they may be in the body. The treatment is usually given in cycles, with periods of rest in between to allow the body to recover.

Chemotherapy can cause side effects such as nausea, vomiting, hair loss, fatigue, and an increased risk of infection. These side effects vary depending on the specific drugs used and the individual's response to treatment. Your healthcare team will closely monitor your condition and provide supportive care to manage any side effects that may arise.

3. Targeted Therapy

Targeted therapy is a newer type of non-surgical treatment that specifically targets cancer cells while sparing healthy cells. It works by blocking the growth and spread of cancer cells by interfering with specific molecules involved in tumor growth. Targeted therapy drugs are usually taken orally.

One type of targeted therapy used for head and neck cancer is cetuximab (Erbitux). It is an antibody that targets a protein called epidermal growth factor receptor (EGFR), which is often overexpressed in head and neck cancer cells. By blocking EGFR, cetuximab can slow down the growth of cancer cells and improve treatment outcomes.

Targeted therapy can have side effects such as skin rash, diarrhea, and infusion reactions. These side effects are usually manageable and temporary. Your healthcare team will closely monitor your condition and provide a guide on how to manage any side effects that may occur.

4. Immunotherapy

Immunotherapy is a promising non-surgical treatment option for head and neck cancer. It works by stimulating the body's immune system to recognize and attack cancer cells. Immunotherapy drugs, such as pembrolizumab (Keytruda) and nivolumab (Opdivo), have shown significant benefits in the treatment of advanced head and neck cancer.

These drugs work by blocking proteins that prevent immune cells from recognizing and attacking cancer cells. By removing this inhibition, immunotherapy helps the immune system better target and destroy cancer cells. Immunotherapy is usually administered intravenously and can be given alone or in combination with other treatments.

Immunotherapy can have side effects such as fatigue, skin rash, diarrhea, and immune-related adverse events. These side effects are usually manageable with the help of your healthcare team. Regular monitoring and communication with your healthcare provider are essential to ensuring early detection and management of any potential side effects.

5. Palliative Care

Palliative care is an important aspect of non-surgical treatment for head and neck cancer, especially for patients with advanced or recurrent disease. Palliative care focuses on providing relief from symptoms and improving the quality of life for patients and their families. It can be provided alongside curative treatments or as the main approach when a cure is no longer possible.

Palliative care may include pain management, symptom control, emotional support, and assistance with decision-making. It aims to address the physical, emotional, and spiritual needs of patients, helping them to live as comfortably and fully as possible.

Chapter 3

Preparing for Treatment

Building Your Support System

When facing a diagnosis of head and neck cancer, it is crucial to have a strong support system in place. Dealing with cancer can be overwhelming, both physically and emotionally, and having the right people by your side can make a significant difference in your journey towards treatment, recovery, and life after diagnosis.

The Importance of Support

A support system consists of individuals who provide emotional, practical, and sometimes even financial assistance during your cancer journey. They can be family members, friends, healthcare professionals, or support groups.

Having a support system in place can help you navigate the challenges that come with head and neck cancer and provide you with the strength and encouragement you need to face them.

Identifying Your Support Network

Building a support system starts with identifying the people who will be there for you throughout your cancer journey. Here are some key individuals and groups to consider:

- **Family and Friends:** Your immediate family and close friends are often the first people you turn to for support. They can provide emotional support, accompany you to medical appointments, help with household chores, and offer a listening ear when you need to talk. It is important to communicate openly with your loved ones about your needs and how they can best support you.

- **Healthcare Professionals:** Your healthcare team, including doctors, nurses, and other medical professionals, plays a vital role in your support system. They have the expertise to guide you through your treatment options, answer your questions, and address any concerns you may have. Building a strong relationship with your healthcare team can provide you with a sense of security and trust throughout your cancer journey.

- **Support Groups:** Support groups consist of individuals who have experienced or are currently going through similar challenges. Joining a support group can provide you with a sense of belonging and understanding. It allows you to connect with others who can relate to your experiences, share advice, and offer emotional support. Support groups can be found in person or online, and many organizations offer specific groups for head and neck cancer patients.

- **Cancer Organizations and Resources:** There are numerous cancer organizations and resources available that can provide valuable information, support, and resources. These organizations often offer educational materials, online forums, helplines, and assistance with practical matters such as financial support or transportation to medical appointments. Connecting with these organizations can help you access the resources you need and connect with others who have faced similar challenges.

Communicating Your Needs

Once you have identified your support network, it is important to communicate your needs effectively. Here are some tips for effective communication:

- **Be Open and Honest:** Share your thoughts, fears, and concerns with your support system. Being open and honest about your emotions and needs can help them understand how best to support you. It is okay to ask for help when you need it.

- **Provide Specific Instructions:** When asking for assistance, be specific about what you need. Whether it is help with household chores, transportation to medical appointments, or simply someone to talk to, providing clear instructions can make it easier for your support system to assist you.

- **Set Boundaries:** While it is important to lean on your support system, it is also crucial to set boundaries. Communicate your limits and let your loved ones know when you need some time alone or when you are not up for visitors. Respecting your boundaries will help maintain a healthy balance between receiving support and taking care of yourself.

Additional Support Resources

In addition to your personal support system, there are various resources available to help you navigate your cancer journey. Here are a few examples:

- **Social Workers:** Many healthcare facilities have social workers who specialize in providing support to cancer patients. They can help you navigate the healthcare system, connect you with resources, and provide emotional support. Social workers are trained professionals who can assist you in managing the practical and emotional aspects of your cancer journey.

- **Mental Health Professionals:** Cancer can take a toll on your mental well-being, and seeking support from mental health professionals can be beneficial. Therapists, psychologists, or counselors can help you cope with the emotional challenges that come with a cancer diagnosis. They can provide you with tools and strategies to manage stress, anxiety, and depression.

- **Online Communities:** The internet offers a wealth of online communities and forums where you can connect with other individuals facing head and neck cancer. These communities provide a platform to share experiences, ask questions, and offer support. However, it is important to verify the credibility of the information shared online and consult with your healthcare team for accurate medical advice.

Understanding Treatment Side Effects

When it comes to treating head and neck cancer, it's important to understand that the journey to recovery may not always be smooth sailing. While the primary goal of treatment is to eliminate cancer cells and promote healing, it's common for patients to experience side effects along the way.

These side effects can vary depending on the type of treatment received, the individual's overall health, and other factors. In this section, we will explore some of the common treatment side effects that you may encounter and provide strategies for managing them.

Side Effects of Surgery

Surgery is a common treatment option for head and neck cancer, and it can have both short-term and long-term side effects. Immediately after surgery, you may experience pain, swelling, and difficulty swallowing or speaking.

These side effects are typically temporary and can be managed with pain medication and supportive care. It's important to follow your healthcare team's instructions for postoperative care to ensure proper healing.

In some cases, surgery may result in changes to your physical appearance, such as the removal of a portion of your jaw or tongue. These changes can have a significant impact on your self-esteem and body image. It's important to remember that you are not defined by your physical appearance and to seek support from loved ones, support groups, or counseling services if needed.

Side Effects of Radiation Therapy

Radiation therapy is another common treatment modality for head and neck cancer. While it can be highly effective in targeting cancer cells, it can also cause side effects. The most common side effects of radiation therapy include fatigue, skin changes, and difficulty swallowing. These side effects typically occur in the area being treated and may worsen as treatment progresses.

To manage fatigue, it's important to prioritize rest and conserve your energy. Take frequent breaks throughout the day and listen to your body's signals. Engaging in light exercise, such as walking, can also help combat fatigue. Additionally, maintaining a healthy diet and staying hydrated can support your body's energy levels.

Skin changes, such as redness, dryness, and peeling, are common during radiation therapy. It's important to keep the treated area clean and moisturized by using gentle skincare products recommended by your healthcare team. Avoid exposing the treated area to direct sunlight, and protect it with clothing or sunscreen.

Difficulty swallowing, known as dysphagia, can occur due to radiation therapy's impact on the muscles and tissues in the throat. Your healthcare team may recommend specific exercises or a modified diet to help manage this side effect. It's important to communicate any difficulties with swallowing to your healthcare team so they can provide appropriate support and guidance.

Side Effects of Chemotherapy and Targeted Therapy

Chemotherapy and targeted therapy are systemic treatments that can affect the entire body. While these treatments can be effective in killing cancer cells, they can also cause side effects. Common side effects of chemotherapy include nausea, hair loss, and fatigue. Targeted therapy may cause similar side effects, but they are often less severe.

To manage nausea, your healthcare team may prescribe anti-nausea medications or recommend dietary changes, such as eating smaller, more frequent meals. It's important to stay hydrated and consume foods that are easy to digest.

If you experience severe or persistent nausea, it's important to communicate this to your healthcare team so they can adjust your treatment plan accordingly.

Hair loss is a common side effect of chemotherapy, and it can have a significant emotional impact. Consider exploring options such as wigs, scarves, or hats to help you feel more comfortable and confident during this time. Remember that hair loss is temporary, and it will likely start to grow back once treatment is completed.

Fatigue is another common side effect of chemotherapy and targeted therapy. It's important to listen to your body and rest when needed. Engaging in light exercise, such as gentle stretching or walking, can also help combat fatigue. Prioritizing a healthy diet and staying hydrated can support your body's energy levels.

Managing Treatment Side Effects

While treatment side effects can be challenging, there are strategies to help manage them and improve your overall well-being during this time. Here are some tips:

1. **Communicate with your healthcare team:** It's important to maintain open and honest communication with your healthcare team. They

can provide guidance, prescribe medications, or recommend supportive therapies to help manage side effects.

2. **Seek support from loved ones:** Surround yourself with a strong support system of family and friends who can provide emotional support and practical assistance during your treatment journey.

3. **Join support groups:** Connecting with others who have gone through or are going through a similar experience can be incredibly helpful. Support groups provide a safe space to share your feelings, ask questions, and learn from others.

4. **Practice self-care:** Prioritize self-care activities that bring you joy and relaxation. This can include activities such as reading, listening to music, practicing mindfulness or meditation, or engaging in hobbies.

5. **Maintain a healthy lifestyle:** Eating a balanced diet, staying hydrated, and engaging in light exercise can help support your overall well-being during treatment. Consult with your healthcare team for specific dietary recommendations.

Remember, every individual's experience with treatment side effects is unique. It's important to work closely with your healthcare team to develop a personalized plan for managing side effects and promoting your recovery. By understanding and addressing these side effects, you can navigate your treatment journey with resilience and improve your quality of life.

Nutrition and Diet During Treatment

When undergoing treatment for head and neck cancer, maintaining proper nutrition and a healthy diet is crucial. The treatments can take a toll on your body, affecting your appetite, taste, and ability to swallow. However, by making some adjustments and following a few guidelines, you can ensure that you are getting the necessary nutrients to support your recovery and overall well-being.

Importance of Nutrition During Treatment

Good nutrition plays a vital role in supporting your body's ability to heal and recover from the effects of cancer treatment. Adequate nutrition can help minimize treatment-related side effects, maintain your strength, and improve your overall quality of life. It can also help boost your immune system, which is essential for fighting off infections and reducing the risk of complications.

Challenges with Eating During Treatment

During treatment, you may experience various challenges that can affect your ability to eat and maintain a healthy diet. Some common challenges include:

1. **Loss of appetite:** Cancer treatments can cause a loss of appetite, making it difficult to consume enough calories and nutrients.
2. **Changes in taste:** Radiation therapy and chemotherapy can alter your sense of taste, making certain foods taste different or unpleasant.
3. **Difficulty swallowing:** Depending on the location and extent of your cancer, you may experience difficulty swallowing, known as dysphagia. This can make it challenging to eat solid foods.
4. **Dry mouth:** Radiation therapy can cause dry mouth, making it harder to chew and swallow food.

Tips for a Nutritious Diet During Treatment

While it may be challenging, it is essential to maintain a nutritious diet during your treatment. Here are some tips to help you overcome the challenges and ensure you are getting the necessary nutrients:

1. **Eat small, frequent meals:** Instead of three large meals, try eating smaller, more frequent meals

throughout the day. This can help you consume enough calories and nutrients without feeling overwhelmed.

2. **Choose nutrient-dense foods:** Choose foods that are packed with nutrients, such as fruits, vegetables, whole grains, lean proteins, and healthy fats. These foods provide essential vitamins, minerals, and antioxidants to support your healing process.

3. **Stay hydrated:** Drink plenty of fluids to stay hydrated, especially if you are experiencing dry mouth. Sip on water, herbal teas, and clear broths throughout the day. Avoid sugary drinks and caffeine, as they can further contribute to dehydration.

4. **Experiment with flavors:** If you are experiencing changes in taste, try experimenting with different flavors and seasonings to make your meals more appealing. Adding herbs, spices, and marinades can help enhance the taste of your food.

5. **Modify food textures:** If you have difficulty swallowing, modify the texture of your food to make it easier to eat. Puree or blend foods to create smooth textures, or choose soft foods that are easier to chew and swallow.

6. **Consider nutritional supplements:** If you are struggling to meet your nutritional needs through food alone, talk to your healthcare team about the possibility of incorporating nutritional supplements into your diet. These supplements can provide additional calories and nutrients to support your recovery.

7. **Manage side effects:** Some treatments may cause side effects that affect your ability to eat. For example, if you are experiencing nausea or vomiting, try eating smaller, more frequent meals and avoiding foods with strong odors. If you have mouth sores, opt for softer foods and avoid spicy or acidic foods that may irritate your mouth.

8. **Seek guidance from a registered dietitian:** A registered dietitian can provide personalized guidance and create a meal plan tailored to your specific needs and challenges. They can help you navigate through the dietary changes and ensure you are getting the right balance of nutrients.

Maintaining proper nutrition and a healthy diet during head and neck cancer treatment is essential for supporting your recovery and overall well-being. Despite the challenges you may face, there are various strategies you can employ to ensure you are getting the necessary nutrients.

By eating small, frequent meals, choosing nutrient-dense foods, staying hydrated, and seeking guidance from a registered dietitian, you can optimize your nutrition and enhance your body's ability to heal. Remember, every small step you take towards a healthy diet can make a significant difference in your treatment journey.

Maintaining Emotional Well-being

Being diagnosed with head and neck cancer can be an overwhelming and emotionally challenging experience. It is important to prioritize your emotional well-being throughout your treatment and recovery journey. Maintaining a positive mindset and finding healthy coping mechanisms can greatly contribute to your overall well-being and enhance your ability to navigate the challenges that lie ahead.

Acknowledge and Express Your Emotions

It is completely normal to experience a wide range of emotions following a cancer diagnosis. You might feel scared, angry, sad, or even guilty. It is important to acknowledge and accept these emotions rather than suppress them. Allow yourself to feel and express your emotions in a healthy manner. Talking to a trusted friend or family member, joining a support group, or seeking professional counseling could all be helpful. You should always feel free to ask for help if you need it.

Seek Support from Loved Ones

Building a strong support system is crucial during your cancer journey. Reach out to your loved ones and let them know how they can support you. Whether it's through emotional support, accompanying you to medical appointments, or simply being there to listen, having a network of people who care about you can make a significant difference in your emotional well-being. Don't hesitate to lean on your support system when you need it most.

Practice Self-Care

Taking care of yourself is essential during this challenging time. Make self-care a priority by engaging in activities that bring you joy and relaxation. This could include hobbies, exercise, meditation, or spending time in nature. Find what works best for you and make time for it regularly. Remember, self-care is not selfish; it is necessary for your overall well-being.

Stay Informed, but Limit Exposure to Negative Information

While it is important to stay informed about your diagnosis and treatment, it is equally important to limit your exposure to negative information. The internet can be a valuable resource, but it can also be overwhelming and filled with misinformation. Stick to reputable sources and avoid spending excessive time researching your condition. Instead, concentrate on the information provided by your healthcare team and put your trust in their knowledge.

Practice Mindfulness and Stress Reduction Techniques

Mindfulness and stress reduction techniques can help you manage anxiety and promote emotional well-being. Consider incorporating practices such as deep breathing exercises, meditation, yoga, or tai chi into your daily routine. These techniques can help you stay present, reduce stress, and improve your overall mental health.

Connect with Others Going Through Similar Experiences

Joining a support group or connecting with others who are going through a similar experience can provide a sense of belonging and understanding. Hearing others' stories and sharing your own can be therapeutic and help you feel less alone. Support groups can be found online or in person, and they offer a safe space to discuss your concerns, ask questions, and gain valuable insights from others who have walked a similar path.

Consider Professional Counseling

If you find that your emotions are becoming overwhelming or interfering with your daily life, seeking professional counseling can be beneficial. A trained therapist can provide you with the tools and support you need to navigate the emotional challenges of your cancer journey. They can help you develop coping strategies, manage anxiety and depression, and provide a safe space for you to express your feelings.

Embrace Positivity and Gratitude

Maintaining a positive mindset can have a profound impact on your emotional well-being. While it is natural to have moments of negativity, try to focus on the positive aspects of your life. Practice gratitude by acknowledging and appreciating the things you are grateful for each day. Surround yourself with positive influences, whether it's uplifting books, music, or spending time with loved ones who bring you joy.

Celebrate Milestones and Achievements

Throughout your treatment and recovery, it is important to celebrate milestones and achievements, no matter how small they may seem. Each step forward is a victory worth acknowledging. Whether it's completing a round of treatment, reaching a personal goal, or simply getting through a difficult day, take the time to recognize and celebrate your accomplishments. This can boost your morale and provide a sense of accomplishment and motivation.

Be Patient with Yourself

Remember to be patient with yourself throughout your cancer journey. Healing takes time, both physically and emotionally. Allow yourself to grieve, to feel, and to heal at your own pace. It is okay to have good days and bad days. Permit yourself to rest when you need it and to ask for help when necessary. Be kind and compassionate to yourself, and remember that you are doing the best you can.

Maintaining your emotional well-being is an ongoing process that requires self-care, support, and a positive mindset. By prioritizing your emotional health, you can navigate the challenges of head and neck cancer with resilience and strength.

Chapter 4

Treatment and Recovery

Surgery and Hospital Stay

Surgery is a common treatment option for head and neck cancer. It involves the removal of the tumor and surrounding tissues to eliminate the cancer cells. The specific surgical procedure will depend on the location and stage of the cancer, as well as the overall health of the patient. In this section, we will explore the different types of surgeries for head and neck cancer and what to expect during your hospital stay.

Types of Surgeries for Head and Neck Cancer

Several types of surgeries may be performed to treat head and neck cancer. The choice of surgery will depend on various factors, including the size and location of the tumor, the stage of the cancer, and the overall health of the patient. Here are some common surgical procedures used in the treatment of head and neck cancer:

1. **Laser Surgery:** This minimally invasive procedure uses a laser beam to remove the tumor. It is often used for small tumors located on the surface of the skin or mucous membranes.

2. **Endoscopic Surgery:** In this procedure, a thin, flexible tube with a camera and surgical instruments is inserted through small incisions to remove the tumor. Endoscopic surgery is commonly used for tumors located in the throat or voice box.

3. **Transoral Robotic Surgery (TORS):** TORS is a minimally invasive procedure that uses a robotic system to remove tumors located in the mouth, throat, or voice box. It offers improved precision and a faster recovery compared to traditional open surgery.

4. **Neck Dissection:** This surgery involves the removal of lymph nodes in the neck to determine if the cancer has spread. It is often performed in conjunction with the removal of the primary tumor.

5. **Glossectomy:** A glossectomy is the surgical removal of all or part of the tongue. It may be necessary for tumors located in the tongue that cannot be treated with less invasive procedures.

6. **Laryngectomy:** This surgery involves the removal of the voice box. It is typically performed for advanced tumors in the larynx that cannot be treated with other methods.

7. **Maxillectomy:** A maxillectomy is the removal of all or part of the upper jawbone. It may be necessary for tumors located in the upper jaw or sinus cavity.

What to Expect During Your Hospital Stay

Undergoing surgery for head and neck cancer will require a hospital stay. The length of your stay will depend on the type of surgery performed and your recovery progress. Here are some things you can expect during your hospital stay:

1. **Preparation:** Before your surgery, you will meet with your surgical team to discuss the procedure and address any concerns or questions you may have. You may need to undergo certain tests or imaging scans to ensure you are in optimal health for surgery.

2. **Anesthesia:** Most head and neck cancer surgeries are performed under general anesthesia, which means you will be asleep during the procedure. An

anesthesiologist will administer the anesthesia and monitor your vital signs throughout the surgery.

3. **Surgical Procedure:** The surgical procedure itself will vary depending on the type of surgery being performed. Your surgeon will make incisions, remove the tumor and surrounding tissues, and reconstruct any affected areas if necessary. The length of the surgery will depend on the complexity of the procedure.

4. **Recovery:** After the surgery, you will be taken to a recovery room where you will be closely monitored as you wake up from anesthesia. You may experience some pain or discomfort, which can be managed with pain medication. Your healthcare team will provide instructions on wound care and any dietary restrictions.

5. **Hospital Stay:** The length of your hospital stay will depend on the extent of the surgery and your recovery progress. You may need to stay in the hospital for a few days or longer. During your stay, your healthcare team will monitor your condition, manage any pain or discomfort, and provide support and guidance.

6. **Post-operative Care:** Once you are discharged from the hospital, you will need to follow specific post-operative care instructions provided by your healthcare team. This may include wound care, dietary restrictions, and follow-up appointments. It is important to closely follow these instructions to ensure proper healing and recovery.

7. **Support and Rehabilitation:** Surgery for head and neck cancer can have a significant impact on your physical and emotional well-being. It is important to seek support from your healthcare team as well as from family, friends, and support groups. Rehabilitation, including speech therapy and physical therapy, may also be recommended to help restore function and improve quality of life.

Remember, every individual's experience with surgery and hospital stay may vary. It is important to communicate openly with your healthcare team and ask any questions or concerns you may have. They are there to support you throughout your treatment journey.

Radiation Therapy

Radiation therapy, also known as radiotherapy, is a common treatment option for head and neck cancer. It uses high-energy radiation to target and destroy cancer cells in the affected area. This treatment can be used alone or in combination with other therapies, such as surgery or chemotherapy, depending on the stage and type of cancer.

How Does Radiation Therapy Work?

Radiation therapy works by damaging the DNA of cancer cells, preventing them from growing and dividing. It can be delivered externally or internally, depending on the specific needs of the patient. External beam radiation therapy is the most common type used for head and neck cancer. It involves directing radiation beams from a machine outside the body toward the tumor site.

Planning for Radiation Therapy

Before starting radiation therapy, you will undergo a planning process to ensure accurate and effective treatment. This process involves several steps:

1. **Simulation:** During simulation, you will be positioned on a treatment table in the same position you will be in during each radiation session. Imaging techniques, such as CT scans, will be used to precisely locate the tumor and determine the optimal radiation angles.

2. **Treatment Planning:** Once the tumor is accurately located, a team of radiation oncologists and medical physicists will develop a treatment plan. They will determine the appropriate radiation dose, the number of treatment sessions, and the angles at which the radiation beams will be delivered.

3. **Customized Devices:** In some cases, customized devices, such as immobilization masks or headrests, may be created to help you maintain the same position during each treatment session. These devices ensure that the radiation beams are consistently targeted at the tumor site.

What to Expect During Radiation Therapy

Radiation therapy is typically delivered in daily sessions over several weeks. Each session lasts only a few minutes, but the entire process can take several weeks to complete. Here's what you can expect during radiation therapy:

1. **Treatment Sessions:** You will be positioned on the treatment table, and the radiation therapist will ensure that you are in the correct position. The radiation machine will then deliver the radiation beams to the targeted area. You will not feel any

pain during the treatment, but you may hear the machine buzzing or clicking.

2. **Side Effects:** Radiation therapy can cause side effects, which vary depending on the specific treatment area and the dose of radiation. Common side effects include fatigue, skin changes, difficulty swallowing, dry mouth, and changes in taste. Your healthcare team will closely monitor your side effects and provide supportive care to manage them.

3. **Lifestyle Adjustments:** During radiation therapy, you may need to make some lifestyle adjustments to minimize side effects and support your overall well-being. This may include maintaining good oral hygiene, following a specific diet, staying hydrated, and avoiding tobacco and alcohol.

Managing the Side Effects of Radiation Therapy

While radiation therapy can be effective in treating head and neck cancer, it can also cause side effects. Here are some strategies to help manage these side effects:

1. **Fatigue:** Fatigue is a common side effect of radiation therapy. To manage fatigue, it's important to prioritize rest and sleep. Listen to your body and take breaks when needed. Engaging in light

physical activity, such as short walks, can also help combat fatigue.

2. **Skin Changes:** Radiation therapy can cause skin irritation and redness in the treated area. To manage skin changes, it's important to keep the area clean and dry. Avoid exposing the area to extreme temperatures, such as hot water or direct sunlight. Use gentle skincare products recommended by your healthcare team.

3. **Difficulty Swallowing and Dry Mouth:** Radiation therapy can affect the salivary glands, leading to difficulty swallowing and dry mouth. To manage these side effects, try eating soft, moist foods and taking small, frequent sips of water throughout the day. Your healthcare team may also recommend saliva substitutes or medications to alleviate dry mouth.

4. **Changes in Taste:** Radiation therapy can temporarily alter your sense of taste. To manage changes in taste, experiment with different flavors and textures to find more appealing foods. Adding herbs and spices to your meals can also enhance the flavor.

Follow-up Care after Radiation Therapy

After completing radiation therapy, you will require regular follow-up appointments to monitor your progress and manage any long-term side effects. These appointments may include physical examinations, imaging tests, and blood work. Your healthcare team will work closely with you to develop a personalized follow-up care plan.

Radiation therapy is a crucial component in the treatment of head and neck cancer. While it can cause side effects, these can often be managed with the help of your healthcare team. By understanding what to expect during radiation therapy and how to manage potential side effects, you can approach this treatment with confidence and focus on your journey toward recovery.

Chemotherapy and Targeted Therapy

Chemotherapy and targeted therapy are two important treatment options for head and neck cancer. While surgery and radiation therapy are often the primary treatments, chemotherapy, and targeted therapy can play a crucial role in the overall treatment plan. In this section, we will explore what chemotherapy and targeted therapy are, how they work, and what to expect during treatment.

Understanding Chemotherapy

Chemotherapy is a systemic treatment that uses drugs to kill cancer cells throughout the body. Unlike surgery or radiation therapy, which target specific areas, chemotherapy is designed to reach cancer cells that may have spread beyond the primary tumor. It can be administered orally or intravenously, and the drugs travel through the bloodstream to reach cancer cells in different parts of the body.

Chemotherapy drugs work by interfering with the cancer cell's ability to divide and grow. They can also target specific proteins or enzymes that are essential for cancer cell survival. While chemotherapy can be effective in killing cancer cells, it can also affect healthy cells in the body, leading to side effects. The specific drugs used and the duration of treatment will depend on the individual's cancer type, stage, and overall health.

Targeted Therapy: A Precision Approach

Targeted therapy is a more recent development in cancer treatment that focuses on specific molecular targets within cancer cells. Unlike chemotherapy, which affects both cancerous and healthy cells, targeted therapy aims to selectively attack cancer cells while minimizing damage to normal cells. This precision approach is made possible by identifying specific genetic or molecular abnormalities that are unique to cancer cells.

Targeted therapy drugs are designed to block the growth and spread of cancer cells by interfering with specific molecules or pathways involved in their development. By targeting these specific abnormalities, targeted therapy can be more effective and have fewer side effects compared to traditional chemotherapy. However, it is important to note that targeted therapy is not suitable for all types of head and neck cancer, and its use depends on the specific molecular characteristics of the tumor.

Combination Therapy: Maximizing Treatment Effectiveness

In some cases, chemotherapy and targeted therapy may be used together or in combination with other treatments like surgery or radiation therapy. This approach, known as combination therapy, aims to maximize the effectiveness of treatment by attacking cancer cells through different mechanisms.

Combination therapy can be particularly beneficial for advanced or recurrent head and neck cancer, where the disease may have spread to other parts of the body. By using multiple treatment modalities, doctors can target cancer cells from different angles, increasing the chances of a successful outcome. However, it is important to note that combination therapy may also increase the risk of side effects as the body is exposed to multiple treatment agents simultaneously.

What to Expect During Chemotherapy and Targeted Therapy

Chemotherapy and targeted therapy are typically administered in cycles, with each cycle consisting of a treatment period followed by a rest period. The duration and frequency of treatment cycles will depend on the specific drugs used and the individual's response to treatment. Treatment may be given in an outpatient setting or in the hospital, depending on the intensity and duration of the therapy.

During chemotherapy, you may experience side effects such as fatigue, nausea, hair loss, and changes in appetite. These side effects are usually temporary and can be managed with medications and lifestyle adjustments. It is important to communicate any side effects to your healthcare team so that they can provide appropriate support and guidance.

Targeted therapy, on the other hand, may have different side effects depending on the specific drugs used. Some common side effects include skin rashes, diarrhea, and high blood pressure. Your healthcare team will closely monitor your response to targeted therapy and adjust the treatment plan as needed.

The Role of Chemotherapy and Targeted Therapy in Head and Neck Cancer

Chemotherapy and targeted therapy can play a crucial role in the treatment of head and neck cancer. They can be used as primary treatments, especially in cases where surgery or radiation therapy may not be feasible. Additionally, they can be used as adjuvant therapies to enhance the effectiveness of other treatments or to target cancer cells that may have spread beyond the primary tumor.

It is important to remember that every individual's treatment plan is unique, and the decision to use chemotherapy or targeted therapy will depend on various factors, including the type and stage of cancer, overall health, and individual preferences. Your healthcare team will work closely with you to determine the most appropriate treatment approach for your specific situation.

In the next section, we will explore the role of rehabilitation and physical therapy in the recovery process after head and neck cancer treatment.

Rehabilitation and Physical Therapy

Rehabilitation and physical therapy play a crucial role in the treatment and recovery process for individuals with head and neck cancer. These therapies aim to restore and improve physical function, reduce pain, and enhance overall quality of life. In this section, we will explore the importance of rehabilitation and physical therapy, the various techniques and exercises involved, and how they can benefit patients during and after treatment.

The Importance of Rehabilitation and Physical Therapy

Head and neck cancer and its treatments can have a significant impact on a person's physical well-being. Surgery, radiation therapy, and chemotherapy can cause a range of side effects, including pain, stiffness, weakness, and difficulty swallowing or speaking. Rehabilitation and physical therapy can help address these issues and improve functional abilities.

One of the primary goals of rehabilitation is to restore and maintain mobility and strength. Physical therapists work closely with patients to develop personalized exercise programs that target specific areas affected by cancer treatment. These exercises may include stretching, strengthening, and range-of-motion exercises to improve flexibility and reduce muscle tightness.

Physical therapy can also help manage pain and discomfort. Therapists may use techniques such as manual therapy, heat or cold therapy, and electrical stimulation to alleviate pain and promote healing. Additionally, they can also provide the needed guide on proper body mechanics and posture to prevent further strain or injury.

Techniques and Exercises

Rehabilitation and physical therapy for head and neck cancer patients involve a variety of techniques and exercises tailored to individual needs. Here are some common approaches used:

1. **Swallowing Therapy:** Many individuals with head and neck cancer experience difficulty swallowing, a condition known as dysphagia. Swallowing therapy, also known as dysphagia therapy, focuses on improving swallowing function and reducing the

risk of aspiration. Therapists may use exercises to strengthen the muscles involved in swallowing, as well as techniques to improve coordination and control.

2. **Speech Therapy:** Speech therapy is essential for patients who have undergone surgery or radiation therapy that affects the structures involved in speech production. Speech therapists can help individuals regain or improve their ability to speak clearly and effectively. Techniques may include vocal exercises, breathing exercises, and strategies to improve articulation and voice projection.

3. **Lymphedema Management:** Lymphedema is a common side effect of head and neck cancer treatment, particularly when lymph nodes are removed or damaged. Physical therapists trained in lymphedema management can also provide guidance on self-care techniques, such as manual lymphatic drainage and compression therapy, to reduce swelling and improve lymphatic flow.

4. **Neck and Shoulder Exercises:** Surgery and radiation therapy can cause stiffness and weakness in the neck and shoulder muscles. Physical therapists can prescribe exercises to improve range

of motion, strengthen muscles, and reduce pain. These exercises may include gentle stretches, resistance training, and postural exercises.

5. **Balance and Coordination Training:** Some individuals may experience balance and coordination issues as a result of treatment. Physical therapists can design exercises to improve balance and coordination, reducing the risk of falls and enhancing overall mobility. These exercises may involve standing on one leg, walking on uneven surfaces, or using specialized equipment to challenge balance.

Benefits of Rehabilitation and Physical Therapy

Engaging in rehabilitation and physical therapy can offer numerous benefits for individuals with head and neck cancer. Some of these benefits include:

1. **Improved Function and Quality of Life:** By addressing physical limitations and reducing pain, rehabilitation, and physical therapy can help individuals regain independence and improve their overall quality of life. Improved mobility, strength, and endurance can enhance daily activities and participation in social and recreational pursuits.

2. **Enhanced Swallowing and Speech Abilities:** Swallowing and speech therapy can significantly improve a person's ability to eat, drink, and communicate effectively. These therapies can help individuals regain confidence in their ability to swallow safely and express themselves clearly.

3. **Pain Management:** Physical therapy techniques, such as manual therapy and therapeutic exercises, can help manage the pain and discomfort associated with head and neck cancer treatment. By addressing the underlying causes of pain, physical therapy can reduce reliance on pain medications and improve overall well-being.

4. **Prevention of Complications:** Rehabilitation and physical therapy can help prevent complications that may arise from treatment, such as lymphedema or muscle contractures. By addressing these issues early on, therapists can minimize the impact on a person's daily life and promote optimal recovery.

Rehabilitation and physical therapy are integral components of the treatment and recovery process for individuals with head and neck cancer. These therapies can help restore physical function, manage pain, and improve overall quality of life.

Chapter 5

Life After Treatment

Follow-up Care and Monitoring

Once you have completed your treatment for head and neck cancer, it is important to continue with regular follow-up care and monitoring. This ongoing care is crucial for detecting any potential recurrence or new cancerous growths, as well as managing any long-term side effects that may arise. In this section, we will discuss the importance of follow-up care, what to expect during follow-up appointments, and how to take an active role in your monitoring and recovery.

The Importance of Follow-up Care

Follow-up care plays a vital role in ensuring your long-term health and well-being after head and neck cancer treatment. Regular check-ups and monitoring allow your healthcare team to closely monitor your progress, detect any signs of recurrence or new cancerous growths, and address any lingering side effects or complications. By staying vigilant and proactive in your follow-up care, you can catch any potential issues early on and increase your chances of successful treatment.

What to Expect During Follow-up Appointments

During your follow-up appointments, your healthcare team will conduct a thorough examination to assess your overall health and monitor for any signs of recurrence or complications. This may include a physical examination of your head and neck area as well as imaging tests such as CT scans or PET scans to get a detailed view of any potential abnormalities. Blood tests may also be conducted to check for any changes in your blood cell counts or tumor markers.

In addition to the physical examination and imaging tests, your healthcare team will also discuss any symptoms or concerns you may have and provide guidance on managing any long-term side effects. They may also refer you to other specialists, such as speech therapists or nutritionists, to address specific issues related to your treatment.

Taking an Active Role in Your Monitoring and Recovery

While your healthcare team will play a crucial role in monitoring your health, you need to take an active role in your monitoring and recovery as well. Here are some steps you can take to ensure you are actively involved in your follow-up care:

1. **Keep a record of your symptoms:** Note down any new or persistent symptoms you experience between appointments. This will help you provide accurate information to your healthcare team and ensure that any potential issues are addressed promptly.

2. **Attend all follow-up appointments:** Make sure to attend all scheduled follow-up appointments, even if you are feeling well. Regular monitoring is essential for detecting any early signs of recurrence or complications.

3. **Communicate openly with your healthcare team:** Be open and honest with your healthcare team about any concerns or questions you may have. They are there to support you and provide guidance throughout your recovery journey.

4. **Maintain a healthy lifestyle:** Adopting a healthy lifestyle can greatly contribute to your overall well-being and reduce the risk of recurrence. This includes eating a balanced diet, engaging in regular physical activity, avoiding tobacco and excessive

    alcohol consumption, and practicing good oral hygiene.

5. **Stay informed:** Educate yourself about the potential long-term side effects of your treatment and how to manage them. This will empower you to take proactive steps toward addressing any issues that may arise.

Frequency of Follow-up Appointments

The frequency of your follow-up appointments will depend on various factors, including the type and stage of your cancer, the treatments you received, and your overall health. In the initial months following treatment, appointments may be more frequent, gradually decreasing in frequency over time. Your healthcare team will determine the appropriate schedule for your follow-up appointments and adjust it as needed based on your circumstances.

Follow-up care and monitoring are essential components of your journey towards conquering head and neck cancer. By actively participating in your monitoring and recovery, attending regular follow-up appointments, and maintaining a healthy lifestyle, you can increase your chances of detecting any potential issues early on and ensuring your long-term well-being. Remember, you are not alone in this journey, and your healthcare team is there to support you every step of the way.

Managing Long-term Side Effects

Managing long-term side effects is an important aspect of life after head and neck cancer treatment. While the primary goal of treatment is to eliminate the cancer and promote recovery, it is common for survivors to experience lingering side effects that can impact their quality of life.

These side effects can vary depending on the type of treatment received and the individual's overall health. In this section, we will explore some of the common long-term side effects and discuss strategies for managing them.

Dental and Oral Health

One of the most common long-term side effects of head and neck cancer treatment is dental and oral health issues. Radiation therapy and certain chemotherapy drugs can cause damage to the teeth, gums, and salivary glands. This can lead to tooth decay, gum disease, dry mouth, and difficulty swallowing.

To manage these side effects, it is important to maintain good oral hygiene practices. Regular dental check-ups and cleanings are essential to monitor and address any dental issues. Your dentist may recommend fluoride treatments or the use of special mouth rinses to help prevent tooth decay. It is also important to stay hydrated and practice good oral hygiene by brushing and flossing regularly.

Swallowing and Eating Difficulties

Another common long-term side effect of head and neck cancer treatment is difficulty swallowing and eating. This can be caused by damage to the muscles and tissues in the throat and esophagus. It can result in pain, discomfort, and a decreased ability to eat and drink normally.

To manage swallowing and eating difficulties, it is important to work with a speech-language pathologist and a dietitian. They can provide exercises and techniques to improve swallowing function and recommend modifications to your diet to make eating easier. This may include eating smaller, more frequent meals, avoiding certain foods that are difficult to swallow, and using thickening agents to make liquids easier to swallow.

Lymphedema

Lymphedema is a condition that can occur as a result of damage to the lymph nodes during head and neck cancer treatment. It is characterized by swelling in the face, neck, or other areas of the body. Lymphedema can be uncomfortable and affect mobility and daily activities.

To manage lymphedema, it is important to work with a lymphedema therapist who can provide specialized techniques to reduce swelling and improve lymphatic flow. This may include manual lymphatic drainage, compression therapy, and exercises to promote circulation. It is also important to practice good skin care and avoid activities that can increase the risk of infection.

Fatigue

Many survivors of head and neck cancer experience fatigue as a long-term side effect. This can be due to a variety of factors, such as the physical and emotional burden of treatment, alterations in sleep patterns, and the impact of specific medications.

To manage fatigue, it is important to prioritize rest. This may involve taking short naps during the day, practicing relaxation techniques such as deep breathing or meditation, and engaging in gentle exercises such as walking or yoga.

It is also important to maintain a balanced diet and stay hydrated to support energy levels.

Emotional and Psychological Effects

The emotional and psychological effects of head and neck cancer can be long-lasting. Many survivors experience anxiety, depression, and changes in body image and self-esteem. It is important to address these issues and seek support from healthcare professionals, support groups, and loved ones.

To manage the emotional and psychological effects, it is important to prioritize self-care and seek professional help if needed. This may involve talking to a therapist or counselor who specializes in cancer survivorship, participating in support groups or counseling sessions, and engaging in activities that bring joy and relaxation.

Long-term Monitoring and Follow-up Care

Regular monitoring and follow-up care are essential for managing long-term side effects and detecting any potential recurrence or new cancer. It is important to attend all scheduled appointments with your healthcare team and communicate any new or persistent symptoms.

During follow-up visits, your healthcare team may perform physical exams, imaging tests, and blood work to monitor your health. They can also provide a guide on managing long-term side effects and address any concerns or questions you may have.

Remember, managing long-term side effects is a journey that requires patience and perseverance. It is important to advocate for yourself and seek support from healthcare professionals, loved ones, and fellow survivors. By taking an active role in your care and making healthy lifestyle choices, you can improve your overall well-being.

Emotional and Psychological Recovery

Dealing with a head and neck cancer diagnosis and undergoing treatment can take a toll not only on your physical well-being but also on your emotional and psychological state. It is completely normal to experience a wide range of emotions during this challenging time. Understanding and addressing these emotions is an essential part of your overall recovery process.

The Emotional Rollercoaster

A head and neck cancer diagnosis can trigger a rollercoaster of emotions. You may feel overwhelmed, scared, angry, or even numb. It is important to remember that these emotions are valid and that it is okay to feel this way. Acknowledging and accepting your emotions is the first step towards emotional and psychological recovery.

Seeking Support

During this time, it is crucial to build a strong support system around you. Reach out to your loved ones, friends, and family members who can provide emotional support. They can be a listening ear, a shoulder to lean on, or even help with practical matters. Don't hesitate to ask for help when you need it.

In addition to your support network, consider joining a support group specifically for head and neck cancer patients. These groups provide a safe space to share experiences, concerns, and emotions with others who have gone through or are going through a similar journey. Hearing from others who have faced similar challenges can be incredibly comforting and empowering.

Professional Help

Sometimes, the emotional and psychological impact of a head and neck cancer diagnosis may require professional help. Don't hesitate to seek the assistance of a mental health professional, such as a therapist or counselor, who specializes in cancer-related issues. They can provide you with the tools and strategies to cope with your emotions and help you navigate through this difficult time.

Coping Strategies

Various coping strategies can help you manage your emotions and promote emotional well-being during your recovery process. Here are a few techniques you may find helpful:

1. **Express Yourself:** Find healthy outlets to express your emotions, such as journaling, painting, or playing a musical instrument. Engaging in creative activities can be therapeutic and provide a sense of release.

2. **Practice Mindfulness:** Incorporate mindfulness techniques into your daily routine. This can include deep breathing exercises, meditation, or yoga. These practices can help you stay present, reduce anxiety, and promote a sense of calm.

3. **Stay Active:** Engaging in regular physical activity can have a positive impact on your emotional well-being. Exercise releases endorphins, which are natural mood boosters. Find activities that you enjoy and make them a part of your routine.

4. **Connect with Nature:** Spending time in nature can have a calming effect on your mind and body. Take walks in the park, sit by the beach, or simply spend time in your garden. Connecting with nature can provide a sense of peace and tranquility.

5. **Educate Yourself:** Knowledge is power. Educate yourself about your diagnosis, treatment options, and potential side effects. Understanding what to expect can help alleviate anxiety and empower you to make informed decisions about your care.

Dealing with Body Image Changes

Head and neck cancer treatments can often result in physical changes that may impact your self-esteem and body image. These changes can include hair loss, scarring, changes in speech or swallowing, and alterations in facial appearance. It is important to remember that these changes do not define your worth or who you are as a person.

If you are struggling with body image issues, consider seeking support from a counselor or therapist who specializes in body image concerns. They can help you navigate through these challenges and develop strategies to improve your self-confidence and acceptance.

Celebrating Milestones

As you progress through your recovery journey, it is important to celebrate milestones, no matter how small they may seem. Each step forward is a victory and a testament to your strength and resilience. Whether it's completing a round of treatment, reaching a specific recovery goal, or simply having a good day, take the time to acknowledge and celebrate these achievements.

Moving Forward

Emotional and psychological recovery is an ongoing process that may continue even after your treatment is complete. Be patient with yourself and allow yourself the time and space to heal emotionally. Remember that you are not alone in this journey, and there is support available to help you navigate through the challenges that may arise.

In the next section, we will explore the importance of support groups and resources that can further assist you in your recovery and provide you with the tools to thrive in your life after treatment.

Support Groups and Resources

Dealing with head and neck cancer can be a challenging journey, both physically and emotionally. It is important to remember that you are not alone in this battle. Support groups and resources can provide you with the guidance, understanding, and encouragement you need to navigate through the various stages of your cancer journey. In this section, we will explore the benefits of support groups and highlight some valuable resources that can assist you in your recovery.

The Power of Support Groups

Support groups play a crucial role in the healing process for individuals facing head and neck cancer. These groups provide a safe and understanding environment where you can connect with others who have gone through similar experiences. Here are some key benefits of joining a support group:

1. **Emotional Support:** Support groups offer a space where you can express your fears, frustrations, and emotions without judgment. Sharing your feelings with others who truly understand can provide immense relief and comfort.

2. **Information and Education**: Support groups often invite healthcare professionals and experts to share valuable information about treatment options, managing side effects, and coping strategies. This

knowledge can empower you to make informed decisions about your health.

3. **Practical Advice:** Members of support groups can offer practical advice based on their own experiences. From tips on managing side effects to recommendations for healthcare providers, these insights can be invaluable in navigating the challenges of treatment and recovery.

4. **Sense of Belonging:** Connecting with others who have faced similar challenges can help combat feelings of isolation. Support groups provide a sense of belonging and a reminder that you are not alone in your journey.

5. **Hope and Inspiration:** Witnessing the resilience and strength of others who have overcome head and neck cancer can provide hope and inspiration during difficult times. Hearing success stories can motivate you to keep fighting and maintain a positive outlook.

Finding the Right Support Group

When searching for a support group, it is important to find one that meets your specific needs and preferences. Here are some tips to help you find the right support group for you:

1. **Ask Your Healthcare Team:** Your healthcare team can be an excellent resource for finding local support groups. They may have connections with organizations or be aware of groups specifically tailored to head and neck cancer patients.

2. **Online Support Groups:** In addition to in-person support groups, there are numerous online communities and forums where you can connect with others facing head and neck cancer. These virtual support groups can be particularly helpful if you are unable to attend in-person meetings or prefer the convenience of online interaction.

3. **Cancer Organizations:** Many cancer organizations offer support groups for individuals with specific types of cancer. Reach out to organizations such as the American Cancer Society, CancerCare, or the Head and Neck Cancer Alliance to inquire about support groups in your area.

4. **Local Hospitals and Treatment Centers:** Hospitals and treatment centers often host support groups for cancer patients. Contact your local healthcare facilities to inquire about any available support groups or resources.

Remember, it may take some time to find the right support group that aligns with your needs and preferences. Don't be discouraged if the first group you try doesn't feel like the right fit. Keep exploring until you find a supportive community that resonates with you.

Additional Resources

In addition to support groups, there are various resources available to assist you in your journey with head and neck cancer. Here are some valuable resources worth exploring:

1. **Cancer Navigators:** Cancer navigators are professionals who can guide you through the complexities of your cancer journey. They can provide information, connect you with resources, and offer emotional support. Reach out to your healthcare team to inquire about the availability of cancer navigators in your area.

2. **Patient Advocacy Organizations:** Patient advocacy organizations, such as the Head and Neck Cancer Alliance and the Oral Cancer Foundation, offer a wealth of information, resources, and support for individuals affected by head and neck cancer. These organizations can provide educational

materials, access to clinical trials, and assistance in finding healthcare providers.

3. **Counseling and Therapy Services:** Dealing with cancer can take a toll on your mental and emotional well-being. Seeking counseling or therapy services can help you navigate the emotional challenges that come with a cancer diagnosis. Your healthcare team can provide recommendations for mental health professionals experienced in working with cancer patients.

4. **Financial Assistance Programs:** Cancer treatment can be financially burdensome. Many organizations offer financial assistance programs to help alleviate some of the financial stress. Reach out to organizations like CancerCare or the Patient Advocate Foundation to inquire about available resources.

Remember, these resources are meant to complement your medical treatment and provide additional support. It is important to consult with your healthcare team before making any decisions or changes to your treatment plan.

Chapter 6

Coping with Recurrence and Advanced Cancer

Understanding Recurrence and Metastasis

Recurrence and metastasis are two terms that can strike fear into the hearts of cancer survivors. After going through the grueling process of treatment and recovery, the thought of the cancer coming back or spreading to other parts of the body can be overwhelming. In this section, we will delve into the topic of recurrence and metastasis, helping you understand what they mean and how they can be managed.

Recurrence: When Cancer Comes Back

Recurrence refers to the return of cancer after a period of remission. It can happen in the same location where the cancer was initially diagnosed or in nearby tissues. The possibility of recurrence is a reality for many cancer survivors, and it's important to be aware of the signs and symptoms that may indicate its presence.

There are different types of recurrence, including local recurrence, regional recurrence, and distant recurrence. Local recurrence means that the cancer has come back to the same area where it was initially found. Regional recurrence indicates that the cancer has spread to nearby lymph nodes or tissues. Distant recurrence, also known as metastasis, occurs when the cancer has spread to distant organs or tissues, such as the lungs, liver, or bones.

The risk of recurrence varies depending on the type and stage of the cancer, as well as the effectiveness of the initial treatment. Some cancers have a higher likelihood of recurrence than others. For example, certain types of head and neck cancers, such as oral cavity cancer, have a higher risk of recurrence compared to others.

Metastasis: When Cancer Spreads

Metastasis is the process by which cancer cells break away from the primary tumor and spread to other parts of the body through the bloodstream or lymphatic system. It is a serious stage of cancer and often indicates a more advanced disease. When cancer metastasizes, it becomes more difficult to treat and manage.

The spread of cancer cells to distant organs or tissues can cause a range of symptoms, depending on the location of the metastasis. For example, if the cancer has spread to the lungs, you may experience shortness of breath or coughing. If it has spread to the bones, you may experience bone pain or fractures. Metastasis can also affect other organs, such as the liver or brain, leading to a variety of symptoms specific to those areas.

It's important to note that not all cancers metastasize. Some cancers, such as basal cell carcinoma, tend to grow locally and rarely spread to other parts of the body. However, other types of cancer, including certain head and neck cancers, have a higher propensity for metastasis.

Managing Recurrence and Metastasis

The management of recurrence and metastasis depends on several factors, including the type and stage of the cancer, the location of the recurrence or metastasis, and the overall health of the individual. Treatment options for recurrence and metastasis may include surgery, radiation therapy, chemotherapy, targeted therapy, immunotherapy, or a combination of these approaches.

In some cases, surgery may be performed to remove the recurrent tumor or the metastatic lesions. Radiation therapy can also be used to target and destroy cancer cells in the affected area. Chemotherapy, targeted therapy, and immunotherapy are systemic treatments that aim to kill cancer cells throughout the body.

It's important to work closely with your healthcare team to determine the most appropriate treatment plan for your specific situation. They will consider various factors, such as the extent of the recurrence or metastasis, the potential benefits and risks of treatment, and your overall health and preferences.

Embracing a Holistic Approach

Dealing with recurrence and metastasis can be emotionally and physically challenging. It's crucial to take a holistic approach to your well-being during this time. This includes not only addressing the physical aspects of the disease but also taking care of your emotional and mental health.

Seeking support from loved ones, joining support groups, or talking to a therapist can provide a valuable outlet for expressing your feelings and fears. Engaging in activities that bring you joy and relaxation, such as hobbies or meditation, can also help reduce stress and improve your overall well-being.

Additionally, maintaining a healthy lifestyle is essential. Eating a balanced diet, staying physically active, and getting enough rest can support your body's ability to fight the disease and cope with treatment. It's also important to follow your healthcare team's recommendations for follow-up care and monitoring to detect any signs of recurrence or metastasis early.

Hope and Resilience

While the thought of recurrence and metastasis can be daunting, it's important to remember that many people have successfully managed these challenges and continued to live fulfilling lives. Advances in medical treatments and supportive care have improved outcomes for individuals facing recurrence and metastasis.

By staying informed, working closely with your healthcare team, and taking care of your overall well-being, you can navigate the journey of recurrence and metastasis with hope and resilience. Remember, you are not alone in this fight, and there are resources and support available to help you every step of the way.

Treatment Options for Recurrence

Dealing with a recurrence of head and neck cancer can be a challenging and emotional experience. After going through the initial treatment and recovery process, the news of a recurrence can feel devastating. However, it's important to remember that there are still treatment options available to you. In this section, we will explore some of the treatment options for recurrence and discuss how they can help you in your journey to conquer head and neck cancer once again.

Re-evaluating the Situation

When faced with a recurrence, it's crucial to undergo a thorough evaluation to determine the extent and location of the cancer. This evaluation may involve various diagnostic tests, such as imaging scans, biopsies, and blood tests. The results of these tests will help your healthcare team develop an appropriate treatment plan tailored to your specific needs.

Surgery

Surgery is often considered a treatment option for recurrent head and neck cancer, especially if the recurrence is localized and has not spread to other parts of the body. The goal of surgery is to remove the cancerous tissue and any surrounding lymph nodes that may be affected.

Depending on the location and size of the recurrence, your surgeon may perform a partial or complete resection of the affected area. In some cases, reconstructive surgery may also be necessary to restore the appearance and function of the affected structures.

Radiation Therapy

Radiation therapy can be an effective treatment option for recurrent head and neck cancer, particularly if surgery is not feasible or if the recurrence is inoperable. This treatment involves the use of high-energy radiation beams to target and destroy cancer cells.

Radiation therapy can be delivered externally (external beam radiation) or internally (brachytherapy). Your radiation oncologist will determine the most appropriate approach based on the location and size of the recurrence.

Chemotherapy and Targeted Therapy

Chemotherapy and targeted therapy are systemic treatments that can be used to treat recurrent head and neck cancer. Chemotherapy involves the use of drugs that kill cancer cells or prevent their growth, while targeted therapy focuses on specific molecular targets within cancer cells.

These treatments can be administered orally or intravenously and may be used alone or in combination with other treatment modalities. Your medical oncologist will determine the most suitable chemotherapy or targeted therapy regimen based on your circumstances.

Immunotherapy

Immunotherapy is a relatively new treatment option that has shown promising results in the management of recurrent head and neck cancer. This approach harnesses the power of the immune system to recognize and destroy cancer cells.

Immunotherapy drugs, such as checkpoint inhibitors, work by blocking the proteins that prevent immune cells from attacking cancer cells. By doing so, they help to enhance the body's natural defense mechanisms against cancer. Immunotherapy may be used as a standalone treatment or in combination with other therapies.

Clinical Trials

Participating in clinical trials can be an option for individuals with recurrent head and neck cancer. Clinical trials are research studies that evaluate new treatment approaches, drugs, or combinations of therapies. By participating in a clinical trial, you may have access to innovative treatments that are not yet widely available. However, it's important to discuss the potential risks and benefits with your healthcare team before considering this option.

Palliative Care

In cases where the recurrence is advanced and curative treatment options are limited, palliative care becomes an essential part of the treatment plan. Palliative care focuses on providing relief from symptoms, managing pain, and improving the quality of life.

It is not limited to end-of-life care and can be initiated at any stage of the disease. Palliative care specialists work closely with the patient and their loved ones to address physical, emotional, and spiritual needs.

Emotional Support

Dealing with a recurrence of head and neck cancer can take a toll on your emotional well-being. It's important to seek emotional support from friends, family, support groups, or mental health professionals.

They can provide a safe space for you to express your feelings, offer guidance, and help you navigate the challenges that come with a recurrence. Remember, you are not alone in this journey, and reaching out for support is a sign of strength.

Making Informed Decisions

When faced with a recurrence, it's crucial to have open and honest conversations with your healthcare team. They can provide you with the necessary information about the available treatment options, their potential benefits, and their possible side effects. Together, you can make informed decisions about your treatment plan based on your circumstances, preferences, and goals.

Palliative Care and Hospice

When facing a diagnosis of advanced head and neck cancer, it's important to understand that there may come a time when curative treatment options are no longer effective or appropriate. This is where palliative care and hospice can play a crucial role in providing comfort, support, and quality of life for both the patient and their loved ones.

What is Palliative Care?

Palliative care is a specialized medical approach that focuses on providing relief from the symptoms, pain, and stress associated with serious illnesses, including advanced head and neck cancer. The goal of palliative care is to improve the overall quality of life for patients and their families by addressing physical, emotional, and spiritual needs.

Palliative care is not limited to end-of-life care. It can be provided at any stage of the disease, alongside curative treatments, and can continue even if the disease progresses. Palliative care teams typically consist of doctors, nurses, social workers, and other healthcare professionals who work together to provide comprehensive support.

The Role of Palliative Care in Advanced Head and Neck Cancer

For patients with advanced head and neck cancer, palliative care can help manage the symptoms and side effects of the disease and its treatments. This may include pain management, addressing swallowing difficulties, managing respiratory issues, and providing emotional support.

Palliative care teams work closely with the patient's primary oncology team to ensure that the treatment plan aligns with the patient's goals and preferences. They can also help facilitate communication between the patient, their family, and the healthcare team, ensuring that everyone is on the same page and that the patient's wishes are respected.

Palliative Care Services

Palliative care services can be provided in various settings, including hospitals, outpatient clinics, and even in the patient's own home. The specific services offered may vary depending on the patient's needs and the resources available in their community.

Some common services provided by palliative care teams include:

1. **Pain and Symptom Management:** Palliative care teams are skilled in managing pain and other distressing symptoms that may arise from advanced head and neck cancer. They can work with the patient's oncology team to develop a personalized pain management plan that may include medications, physical therapy, and other interventions.

2. **Emotional and Psychological Support:** Dealing with advanced head and neck cancer can take a toll on a patient's emotional well-being. Palliative care teams can provide counseling, support groups, and other resources to help patients and their families cope with the emotional challenges they may face.

3. **Spiritual and Existential Support:** Palliative care recognizes that the emotional and spiritual well-being of patients is just as important as their physical health. Chaplains or other spiritual care providers may be available to offer guidance, comfort, and support to patients and their families, regardless of their religious or spiritual beliefs.

4. **Caregiver Support:** Caring for a loved one with advanced head and neck cancer can be physically and emotionally demanding. Palliative care teams can provide support and resources for caregivers, helping them navigate the challenges they may encounter and ensuring they have the necessary tools to provide the best care possible.

Hospice Care

Hospice care is a specialized form of palliative care that is focused on providing comfort and support to patients who are nearing the end of their lives. Hospice care is typically provided when curative treatments are no longer effective or desired, and the focus shifts to maximizing quality of life.

Hospice care can be provided in various settings, including the patient's home, a hospice facility, or a hospital. The primary goal of hospice care is to ensure that patients are as comfortable and pain-free as possible during their final days, while also providing emotional and spiritual support to both the patient and their loved ones.

Hospice care teams consist of healthcare professionals who are experienced in end-of-life care. They work closely with the patient's primary care team and palliative care team to ensure a seamless transition and continuity of care.

Making Decisions About Palliative Care and Hospice

Deciding to pursue palliative care or hospice is a deeply personal decision that should be made in consultation with the patient, their loved ones, and their healthcare team. It's important to have open and honest conversations about the patient's goals, preferences, and concerns.

Palliative care and hospice can provide invaluable support and comfort during a challenging time. By focusing on the patient's overall well-being and quality of life, these specialized forms of care can help patients and their families navigate the physical, emotional, and spiritual challenges of advanced head and neck cancer.

Living with Advanced Cancer

Living with advanced cancer can be a challenging and emotional journey. As you navigate through this stage of your cancer journey, it's important to remember that you are not alone. There are resources, support systems, and strategies available to help you cope with the physical, emotional, and practical aspects of living with advanced cancer.

Understanding Advanced Cancer

Advanced cancer refers to cancer that has spread from its original site to other parts of the body. This stage of cancer can be overwhelming, as it often comes with a range of physical symptoms and emotional challenges. It's important to have a clear understanding of your diagnosis and prognosis, as this will help you make informed decisions about your treatment and care.

Managing Symptoms and Side Effects

Living with advanced cancer often involves managing a range of symptoms and side effects. These can vary depending on the type and location of your cancer, as well as the treatments you are receiving. It's important to work closely with your healthcare team to develop a personalized symptom management plan. This may include medications, lifestyle changes, and complementary therapies to help alleviate pain, nausea, fatigue, and other symptoms.

Emotional Support and Coping Strategies

Dealing with advanced cancer can take a toll on your emotional well-being. It's normal to experience a range of emotions, including fear, sadness, anger, and anxiety. Seeking emotional support from loved ones, support groups, or mental health professionals can be beneficial. They can provide a safe space for you to express your feelings and offer coping strategies to help you navigate the emotional challenges of living with advanced cancer.

Palliative Care and Hospice

Palliative care focuses on providing relief from the symptoms and stress of a serious illness, such as advanced cancer. It is not limited to end-of-life care and can be provided alongside curative treatments. Palliative care teams work closely with your healthcare team to manage pain, improve quality of life, and provide emotional support.

Hospice care, on the other hand, is specifically designed for individuals with a life expectancy of six months or less. It focuses on providing comfort and support during the end stages of life.

Making the Most of Your Time

Living with advanced cancer can bring a renewed sense of urgency and a desire to make the most of your time. It's important to prioritize activities and experiences that bring you joy and fulfillment. This may include spending quality time with loved ones, pursuing hobbies and interests, or creating meaningful memories. It's also important to take care of yourself physically and emotionally, ensuring you have the energy and strength to engage in activities that are important to you.

Planning for the Future

While living with advanced cancer, it's important to consider your plans and make the necessary arrangements. This may include discussing your wishes for end-of-life care, creating a will or advance directive, and ensuring your financial and legal affairs are in order. Having these conversations and making these arrangements can provide peace of mind and alleviate some of the stress associated with advanced cancer.

Finding Support and Resources

There are numerous support groups, organizations, and resources available to individuals living with advanced cancer. These can provide valuable information, emotional support, and practical assistance. Reach out to local cancer support organizations, online communities, or your healthcare team to find resources that are relevant to your specific needs.

Celebrating Life

Living with advanced cancer is not just about surviving; it's about finding joy and celebrating life. Take the time to appreciate the small moments, find gratitude in everyday experiences, and surround yourself with positivity. Celebrate milestones, achievements, and the strength and resilience you have shown throughout your cancer journey.

Remember, living with advanced cancer is a unique and personal experience. It's important to find what works best for you and to seek support when needed. Embrace the journey, cherish the moments, and continue to live life to the fullest, one day at a time.

Chapter 7

Promoting Prevention and Awareness

Preventing Head and Neck Cancer

Preventing head and neck cancer is a crucial step in reducing the burden of this disease. While not all cases of head and neck cancer can be prevented, there are several measures you can take to lower your risk. In this section, we will discuss some of the key strategies for preventing head and neck cancer.

Avoid Tobacco and Alcohol

One of the most important steps you can take to prevent head and neck cancer is to avoid tobacco and excessive alcohol consumption. Tobacco use, including smoking cigarettes, cigars, and pipes, is a major risk factor for head and neck cancer. It is estimated that up to 85% of head and neck cancers are linked to tobacco use.

Alcohol consumption, especially heavy drinking, also increases the risk of developing head and neck cancer. When combined with tobacco use, the risk is even higher. If you currently smoke or drink alcohol, quitting or reducing your consumption can significantly lower your risk of developing head and neck cancer.

Practice Safe Sex and Reduce HPV Exposure

Human papillomavirus (HPV) is a common sexually transmitted infection that can increase the risk of developing head and neck cancer, particularly oropharyngeal cancer. Engaging in safe sex practices, such as using condoms and limiting the number of sexual partners, can help reduce the risk of HPV infection.

Vaccination against HPV is another effective way to prevent infection and reduce the risk of developing head and neck cancer. The HPV vaccine is recommended for both males and females, ideally before becoming sexually active. Talk to your healthcare provider about the HPV vaccine and whether it is appropriate for you or your children.

Protect Yourself from Sun Exposure

Excessive exposure to the sun's harmful ultraviolet (UV) rays can increase the risk of developing lip and skin cancers, which are types of head and neck cancer. To protect yourself from sun exposure:

- Seek shade when the sun is strongest, usually between 10 a.m. and 4 p.m.
- Wear protective clothing, such as wide-brimmed hats and long-sleeved shirts.
- Use sunscreen with a sun protection factor (SPF) of 30 or higher on exposed skin, and reapply every two hours or after swimming or sweating.
- Wear sunglasses that block both UVA and UVB rays to protect your eyes and the delicate skin around them.

By taking these precautions, you can reduce your risk of developing head and neck cancer related to sun exposure.

Eat a Healthy Diet

Maintaining a healthy diet can also play a role in preventing head and neck cancer. A diet rich in fruits, vegetables, and whole grains provides essential nutrients and antioxidants that help protect against cancer. On the other hand, a diet high in processed foods, red meat, and unhealthy fats may increase the risk of developing cancer.

To promote a healthy diet:

- Include a variety of colorful fruits and vegetables in your meals.
- Choose whole grains, such as brown rice, whole wheat bread, and quinoa.
- Limit the consumption of processed foods, sugary drinks, and red meat.
- Choose lean proteins, such as fish, poultry, and legumes.
- Stay hydrated by drinking plenty of water.

By adopting a healthy eating pattern, you can support your overall health and reduce the risk of developing head and neck cancer.

Practice Good Oral Hygiene

Maintaining good oral hygiene is not only important for your dental health but also for preventing head and neck cancer. Poor oral hygiene can lead to chronic inflammation and infections, which can increase the risk of developing oral cavity and oropharyngeal cancers.

To practice good oral hygiene:

- Brush your teeth at least twice a day with fluoride toothpaste.

- Floss daily to remove plaque and food particles between your teeth.
- Visit your dentist regularly for checkups and cleanings.
- Avoid tobacco products, which can increase the risk of oral cancer.
- Limit alcohol consumption, as excessive drinking is a risk factor for oral cancer.

By taking care of your oral health, you can reduce the risk of developing head and neck cancer and maintain a healthy smile.

Stay Hydrated and Limit Exposure to Environmental Hazards

Staying hydrated is essential for overall health and can also help reduce the risk of developing head and neck cancer. Drinking an adequate amount of water helps keep the mucous membranes in your mouth and throat moist, reducing the risk of irritation and inflammation.

Additionally, it is important to limit exposure to environmental hazards that may increase the risk of head and neck cancer. This includes avoiding prolonged exposure to certain chemicals, such as asbestos, formaldehyde, and certain industrial solvents. If you work in an environment where you may be exposed to these substances, follow safety guidelines and use protective equipment.

Regular Check-ups and Screenings

Regular check-ups with your healthcare provider are crucial for the early detection and prevention of head and neck cancer. During these visits, your healthcare provider can perform a thorough examination of your head and neck, including your mouth, throat, and lymph nodes.

Depending on your risk factors and medical history, your healthcare provider may recommend additional screenings, such as a head and neck cancer screening or an HPV test. These screenings can help detect any abnormalities or early signs of cancer, allowing for prompt treatment and better outcomes.

Preventing head and neck cancer requires a combination of lifestyle changes, regular screenings, and awareness of risk factors. By avoiding tobacco and excessive alcohol consumption, practicing safe sex, protecting yourself from sun exposure, maintaining a healthy diet, practicing good oral hygiene, staying hydrated, and limiting exposure to environmental hazards, you can significantly reduce your risk of developing head and neck cancer.

The Importance of Early Detection

Early detection plays a crucial role in the successful treatment and management of head and neck cancer. Detecting cancer at an early stage can significantly improve the chances of a positive outcome and increase the effectiveness of treatment options. In this section, we will explore why early detection is so important and discuss the various methods available for early detection.

Why is Early Detection Important?

Early detection of head and neck cancer is vital for several reasons. Firstly, it allows for a more targeted and less invasive treatment approach. When cancer is detected at an early stage, it is often localized and has not spread to other parts of the body. This means that treatment can be focused on the affected area, minimizing the need for extensive surgery or aggressive therapies.

Secondly, early detection can lead to a higher chance of a cure. The earlier cancer is diagnosed, the more likely it is to be successfully treated. By catching the disease in its early stages, medical professionals have a better chance of completely removing the cancerous cells and preventing further growth or spread.

Furthermore, early detection can help reduce the physical and emotional burden on patients. Detecting cancer early may allow for less aggressive treatment options, resulting in fewer side effects and a quicker recovery. It can also alleviate the anxiety and uncertainty that often accompany a cancer diagnosis, as patients can take immediate action and begin treatment promptly.

Methods of Early Detection

There are several methods available for the early detection of head and neck cancer. These methods may be used individually or in combination, depending on the specific circumstances and the recommendations of healthcare professionals. Let's explore some of the most common methods:

1. **Regular Self-Examination:** Performing regular self-examinations is a simple yet effective way to detect any changes or abnormalities in the head and neck region. By becoming familiar with the normal appearance and feel of your neck, throat, and mouth, you can quickly identify any unusual lumps, sores, or changes in your voice. If you notice any persistent or concerning symptoms, it is important

to consult a healthcare professional for further evaluation.

2. **Dental Check-ups:** Regular dental check-ups are not only essential for maintaining oral health but also for the early detection of head and neck cancer. During routine dental visits, dentists thoroughly examine the mouth, gums, and throat for any signs of abnormalities. They may also perform additional tests, such as oral brush biopsies, to further investigate suspicious areas. Dental professionals are often the first to detect early signs of oral cancer, making regular dental visits an important part of early detection.

3. **Medical Screenings:** Medical screenings, such as physical examinations and imaging tests, are crucial for the early detection of head and neck cancer. During a physical examination, healthcare professionals may palpate the neck and throat to check for any enlarged lymph nodes or abnormal masses. Imaging tests, such as X-rays, CT scans, or MRIs, can provide detailed images of the head and neck region, allowing for the identification of any tumors or abnormalities.

4. **Biopsies:** If suspicious areas are identified during a physical examination or imaging test, a biopsy may be performed to confirm the presence of cancer cells. A biopsy involves the removal of a small tissue sample from the affected area, which is then examined under a microscope by a pathologist. Biopsies are the most definitive method of diagnosing head and neck cancer and can provide valuable information about the type and stage of the disease.

5. **HPV Testing:** Human papillomavirus (HPV) is a known risk factor for certain types of head and neck cancer. HPV testing can help identify the presence of the virus in the body, which can be an early indicator of potential cancer development. This test is often recommended for individuals with a history of HPV infection or other risk factors.

The Role of Education and Awareness

In addition to individual efforts, education, and awareness play a crucial role in promoting early detection of head and neck cancer. By educating the general public about the signs and symptoms of the disease, individuals are more likely to seek medical attention if they notice any concerning changes in their head and neck region. Public awareness campaigns, community outreach programs, and educational materials can all contribute to increasing knowledge and understanding of head and neck cancer.

Furthermore, healthcare professionals should be well-informed about the latest advancements in early detection methods and guidelines. By staying up-to-date with current research and best practices, they can provide accurate information and guidance to their patients, ultimately improving the chances of early detection and successful treatment.

Raising Awareness and Advocacy

Raising awareness about head and neck cancer is crucial to educate the public, reduce stigma, and promote early detection. Advocacy plays a vital role in ensuring that the needs of head and neck cancer patients are met and that research and innovation continue to advance in the field. In this section, we will explore the importance of raising awareness and advocating for the fight against head and neck cancer.

The Power of Awareness

Raising awareness about head and neck cancer is essential for several reasons. First and foremost, it helps to educate the public about the signs, symptoms, and risk factors associated with the disease. By increasing knowledge and understanding, we can empower individuals to recognize potential warning signs and seek medical attention promptly.

Furthermore, awareness campaigns can help reduce the stigma often associated with head and neck cancer. Many people are unaware of the impact this disease can have on a person's life, including the physical, emotional, and psychological challenges they may face. By shedding light on these issues, we can foster empathy and support for those affected by the disease.

Raising awareness also plays a crucial role in promoting early detection. Early diagnosis is key to successful treatment outcomes, as it allows for more effective intervention and a higher chance of a cure. By encouraging individuals to undergo regular screenings and seek medical attention at the first sign of symptoms, we can improve survival rates and the overall prognosis.

Advocacy for Head and Neck Cancer

Advocacy is an essential component of the fight against head and neck cancer. It involves speaking up for the needs and rights of patients, promoting policy changes, and supporting research and innovation in the field. Advocacy can take many forms, from grassroots initiatives to national and international campaigns.

One of the primary goals of advocacy is to ensure that head and neck cancer patients have access to high-quality care and support. This includes advocating for affordable and comprehensive health insurance coverage as well as promoting the availability of specialized treatment centers and multidisciplinary care teams. By advocating for these resources, we can help improve the overall quality of life for patients and survivors.

Advocacy also plays a crucial role in promoting research and innovation in the field of head and neck cancer. By supporting funding initiatives and raising awareness about the importance of research, we can help drive advancements in treatment options, early detection methods, and supportive care.

Advocacy efforts can also help facilitate collaboration between researchers, clinicians, and patients, leading to more effective and patient-centered approaches to care.

Getting Involved

There are many ways to get involved in raising awareness and advocating for head and neck cancer. Here are a few suggestions:

1. **Join or support advocacy organizations:** There are numerous organizations dedicated to raising awareness and advocating for head and neck cancer patients. Consider joining or supporting these organizations through donations, volunteering, or participating in their events and campaigns.

2. **Share your story:** If you or a loved one has been affected by head and neck cancer, consider sharing your story. Personal narratives can be powerful tools for raising awareness and inspiring others to take action.

3. **Participate in awareness campaigns:** Many organizations and healthcare institutions run awareness campaigns throughout the year. Get involved by sharing information on social media, organizing local events, or participating in fundraising activities.

4. **Contact your elected officials:** Reach out to your local, state, and national representatives to advocate for policies that support head and neck cancer

patients. This can include advocating for increased funding for research, improved access to care, and the inclusion of patient perspectives in healthcare decision-making.

5. **Support research initiatives:** Consider donating to research organizations or participating in clinical trials. By supporting research efforts, you can contribute to the development of new treatments and improved outcomes for head and neck cancer patients.

Remember, every effort, no matter how small, can make a difference in the fight against head and neck cancer. By raising awareness and advocating for change, we can improve the lives of those affected by this disease and work towards a future free from its devastating impact.

Supporting Research and Innovation

Research and innovation play a crucial role in the fight against head and neck cancer. They are the driving forces behind advancements in treatment options, improved outcomes, and ultimately, the quest for a cure. In this section, we will explore the importance of supporting research and innovation in the field of head and neck cancer.

The Need for Research

Head and neck cancer is a complex disease with various subtypes and stages, each requiring tailored treatment approaches. Research helps us better understand the underlying causes, risk factors, and mechanisms of this disease. It allows us to identify new targets for treatment and develop innovative therapies that can improve patient outcomes.

By supporting research, we can uncover new diagnostic tools, treatment modalities, and preventive strategies. This knowledge not only benefits current patients but also future generations by providing them with more effective and less invasive treatment options.

Funding Research

Funding is a critical component in supporting research and innovation. It enables scientists and researchers to conduct studies, gather data, and develop new therapies. There are several ways individuals and organizations can contribute to funding research on head and neck cancer:

1. **Donations:** Making financial contributions to reputable organizations and research institutions dedicated to head and neck cancer research is a direct way to support ongoing studies. These

donations can be made in memory of a loved one, as a tribute to a survivor, or simply as a way to contribute to the advancement of medical science.

2. **Fundraising Events:** Organizing or participating in fundraising events such as walks, runs, or charity auctions can help raise funds for research. These events not only generate financial support but also raise awareness about head and neck cancer and the importance of research.

3. **Corporate Sponsorship:** Companies can play a significant role in supporting research by providing financial support or in-kind donations. By partnering with research institutions or organizations, corporations can contribute to the development of new treatments and technologies.

4. **Grants and Scholarships:** Governments, foundations, and organizations often offer grants and scholarships to researchers and scientists working in the field of head and neck cancer. These grants provide financial support for research projects and help attract talented individuals to the field.

Clinical Trials

Clinical trials are an essential part of the research process. They allow researchers to test new treatments, therapies, and interventions in a controlled environment. Participating in clinical trials not only provides patients with access to cutting-edge treatments but also contributes to the advancement of medical knowledge.

If you are interested in participating in a clinical trial, it is important to discuss this option with your healthcare team. They can provide information about ongoing trials, eligibility criteria, potential risks, and benefits. By participating in a clinical trial, you become an active participant in the search for better treatments and outcomes for head and neck cancer.

Collaboration and Knowledge Sharing

Collaboration and knowledge sharing are vital in the field of head and neck cancer research. By working together, researchers can pool their expertise, resources, and data to accelerate progress. Collaboration can occur between different research institutions, healthcare providers, and even across international borders.

In addition to collaboration, sharing research findings and data is crucial for advancing knowledge in the field.

Open-access journals, conferences, and scientific meetings provide platforms for researchers to present their work and exchange ideas. This sharing of information fosters innovation and allows for the development of new treatment strategies.

Advocacy for Research

Advocacy plays a significant role in supporting research and innovation. By raising awareness about the importance of head and neck cancer research, we can garner public support and encourage policymakers to allocate more funding to this area. Advocacy efforts can include:

1. **Educating the Public:** Spreading awareness about head and neck cancer, its impact, and the need for research can help generate public interest and support. This can be done through educational campaigns, public lectures, and media outreach.

2. **Engaging with Policymakers:** Advocacy groups can work directly with policymakers to highlight the importance of funding research and innovation in head and neck cancer. By sharing personal stories, statistics, and scientific evidence, they can make a compelling case for increased investment.

3. **Supporting Legislation:** Advocacy groups can support or initiate legislation that promotes funding for head and neck cancer research. This can include advocating for increased research budgets, tax incentives for research donations, or policies that prioritize research funding.

The Role of Technology

Technology plays a significant role in advancing research and innovation in head and neck cancer. From medical imaging techniques to genomic sequencing, technological advancements have revolutionized our understanding and treatment of this disease. Some key areas where technology has made an impact include:

1. **Precision Medicine:** Advances in genomic sequencing and molecular profiling have allowed for the development of personalized treatment approaches. By analyzing a patient's genetic makeup, doctors can identify specific mutations or biomarkers that can be targeted with precision therapies.

2. **Imaging and Screening**: Improved imaging techniques such as PET-CT scans and MRI have enhanced our ability to detect and diagnose head

and neck cancer at earlier stages. This early detection can significantly improve treatment outcomes and survival rates.

3. **Robot-Assisted Surgery:** Robotic surgical systems have revolutionized the field of head and neck cancer surgery. These systems provide surgeons with enhanced precision, dexterity, and visualization, resulting in better surgical outcomes and reduced complications.

4. **Telemedicine:** Telemedicine has become increasingly important, especially in the context of remote or underserved areas. It allows patients to access specialized care, consultations, and follow-up appointments without the need for extensive travel.

The Power of Hope

Supporting research and innovation in head and neck cancer is not just about funding and technology; it is also about fostering hope. Every dollar donated, every clinical trial participant, and every research breakthrough brings us one step closer to a future where head and neck cancer is no longer a life-threatening disease.

Conclusion

Living with Hope

As we reach the end of this journey together, I hope that you now feel empowered, supported, and ready to move forward with your head held high. While cancer presents profound challenges, you have the inner strength and resources to meet them.

Trust in your care team, but remember that you are the captain of your treatment plan. This is your life, and your voice matters. Ask questions, express your needs, and lean on your loved ones through the difficult days. You must care for your whole self—body, mind, and spirit.

It won't always be easy, but you now have strategies to navigate every step. Treasure each accomplishment, celebrate small joys, and find meaning in everyday moments. Share your experiences to lift others.

You are defined not by cancer but by your courage, wisdom, and deep resilience. Treatments will continue improving, but your willpower starts now. Believe in your ability to conquer anything. Stay focused on the future, filled with possibilities that await you.

This is not the end, but the beginning of a new chapter. Keep seeking knowledge, embracing hope, and living fully. Continue standing strong. You are ready for whatever comes next, more empowered than ever before.

The journey of a thousand miles begins with a single step. Take that step today.

Isabella White.

www.ingramcontent.com/pod-product-compliance
Lightning Source LLC
Chambersburg PA
CBHW071604270726
48661CB00018B/1240